Using Spirituality in EMDR Therapy

Using Spirituality in EMDR Therapy offers a means for EMDR therapists to integrate a spiritual perspective into their own lives as well as their clinical practice.

The book offers a valuable alternative to traditional forms of psychotherapy by placing an emphasis on purpose and meaning. Taking a spiritually informed model, Heart Led Psychotherapy (HLP), which is applicable to anyone regardless of their spiritual beliefs, the book uses a BioPsychoSocioSpiritual approach to treat psychological distress. The book provides a comprehensive guide on how to incorporate spirituality into each of the 8 phases of EMDR therapy and beyond. It will increase your confidence to work spiritually with clients to deepen their transformative healing process and support them to live a more authentic, heart led life.

Illustrated with case studies to highlight key points and including a range of practical resources, exercises, scripts and strategies, this engaging book will be of great interest to EMDR therapists.

Dr Alexandra Dent is a Registered and Chartered Clinical Psychologist working in independent practice in the UK. Areas of interest include trauma, attachment, mindfulness and spirituality. Alexandra is a Europe accredited EMDR Child and Adolescent Consultant, EMDR Consultant and Training Facilitator. She set up the UK Special Interest Group in EMDR and Spirituality in 2019.

'In her insightful book, Dr Alexandra Dent, developer of Heart Led Psychotherapy (HLP), explores the profound synergy between EMDR and spirituality, elevating EMDR beyond mere symptom reduction. While EMDR is known for its effectiveness in alleviating distress, Dr Dent reveals how integrating spiritual practices can deepen and enhance the healing process. Full of case examples, ways to explain new concepts, and practical tips, this book is perfect for EMDR therapists looking to deepen their practice with clients, demonstrating that EMDR's true potential lies in its ability to foster holistic, transformative growth.'

Rotem Brayer, *approved EMDR Consultant, and author of* The Art and Science of EMDR

'Jung said, "Science works harm only when it is seen as the only thing." We are evidence-based professionals who respect the scientific studies that demonstrate why EMDR is effective. Our patients, however, often see their struggles as spiritual rather than scientific. It is difficult to find books brave enough to combine science with the spiritual. Dr Alexandra Dent has combined both perspectives beautifully. Those interested in expanding beyond science to explore the spiritual aspect that EMDR elicits must read this beautiful book.'

Dr Andrew J. Dobo, *Licensed Psychologist, EMDRIA Approved EMDR Consultant and Trainer. Author of* Unburdening Souls at the Speed of Thought: Psychology, Christianity, and the Transforming power of EMDR *and* The Hero's Journey: Integrating Jungian Psychology and EMDR Therapy

'A beautiful book, from a beautiful soul. Alexandra Dent's highly accessible text expertly guides the reader on this important journey from the EMDR standard protocol to a full BioPsychoSocioSpiritual model.'

Annabel McGoldrick, *PhD of EMDRInsight.com*

'Dr Alexandra Dent has combined both her passion for EMDR and spirituality within this informative work. The book invites EMDR clinicians to consider whether they are working through the lens of ego, or a heart and soul led approach and provides clinical case examples to illustrate her model. A heart and soul led approach is a welcome addition to the field.'

Nic Hartshorne, *Accredited EMDR Clinician, Secretary of the UK EMDR Spirituality Special Interest Group, Chair of the BACP spirituality division*

'Alexandra Dent's Transpersonal Psychology and EMDR delves into the convergence of spiritual and psychological healing. Dent masterfully blends the transformative power of Eye Movement Desensitization and Reprocessing (EMDR) with the rich, expansive principles of transpersonal psychology. She offers a compelling approach for integrating spiritual dimensions into therapeutic practice, providing practitioners with innovative tools to support clients' deeper healing and self-discovery. This book is a valuable resource for therapists, counsellors, and anyone interested in confidently incorporating soul-work into psychology. A definite read for anyone committed to advancing their EMDR practice via expanding their understanding of the human experience, incorporating new tools and returning to the work of psychotherapy as caring for the soul.'

Oraine Ramoo, *EMDR Certified Therapist and EMDRIA Approved Consultant*

Using Spirituality in EMDR Therapy

The Heart Led Approach

Alexandra Dent

Routledge
Taylor & Francis Group

LONDON AND NEW YORK

Designed cover image: Cover image by Amanda Wood, Facebook page: AmandaWoodArts

First published 2025
by Routledge
4 Park Square, Milton Park, Abingdon, Oxon OX14 4RN

and by Routledge
605 Third Avenue, New York, NY 10158

Routledge is an imprint of the Taylor & Francis Group, an informa business

British Library Cataloguing-in-Publication Data
A catalogue record for this book is available from the British Library

ISBN: 978-1-032-83502-0 (hbk)
ISBN: 978-1-032-83499-3 (pbk)
ISBN: 978-1-003-50964-6 (ebk)

DOI: 10.4324/9781003509646

Typeset in Times New Roman
by Taylor & Francis Books

To all that was, is and ever will be,
In Divine love.

Contents

Figures

Preface

'Would you become a pilgrim on the road of love? The first condition is that you make yourself humble as dust and ashes.'

Rumi

The breath is always there as a guide during our life; our point of reference to keep coming back to, to ground ourselves and take a moment's pause. Knowing this has probably been the most valuable and essential tool I have learned during my spiritual journey. Remembering to do this has been a life saver at times, during those intense and often brutal challenges and purges. Learning to connect, heal and deepen the relationship with my heart has been the other critical tool I have had to embrace, because within this space I have direct access to my soul and the Divine. Within my heart I can hear my inner truth, wisdom and authenticity, which stifles out the rumbling energetic and often loud ego in the background. Combining the breath and heart enables one to make different choices, learn important life lessons and heal deep inner wounds which can sometimes be in the form of soul trauma.

I was often told by spiritual healers that I had to 'walk the walk to talk the talk.' I still do! This in reality has meant that I have had to practise what I preach in all areas of my life; to completely surrender and trust my soul and the Divine and remember to keep coming back to my breath and heart, because within that space I am able to find calm and guidance.

And so it is that this book pulls together my experience both in my personal and clinical life to provide you with as many tools and insights as I can, supporting your clients as well as yourself in your spiritual Eye Movement Desensitisation and Reprocessing (EMDR) practice.

My EMDR journey

I can still clearly recall that moment, sitting in the first part of my EMDR training after half an hour in, when my soul felt a huge sense of relief and excitement that I had finally connected with something fundamentally significant for my future clinical work. It was November 2009, the weather was unusually very cold and snowy, so much so that I couldn't travel to the first evening's teaching and I didn't know whether I was going to be able to travel the next day to attend the rest of the training. My ego provided many reasons not to attend, with two young children and a 'busy' life. Yet something guided me from deep within, so I braved the weather and thankfully arrived safely at the hotel where the training was taking place. I sat there, experiencing a huge buzz of excitement, as finally things started making sense. Whilst I had trained in various modalities throughout my Clinical Psychology training, I had never deeply connected with the core traditional models taught. Now I was being shown not only how to formulate from a trauma perspective but about the tools that can actually provide effective intervention. It was very apparent how versatile EMDR could be in response to so many clinical presentations.

Another special moment for me during this EMDR training was when one of the trainers, Michael Paterson, described how to resource clients by connecting them with their auras. This was music to my heart and soul. Up until this point I had felt the need to be careful with the spiritual part of me in my clinical work. I often felt I was working 'undercover' when using aspects of spirituality in sessions, for fear of being found out, reprimanded or sacked. It was a time where spirituality and psychotherapy were still very separate and not encouraged within our work, especially in the National Health Service (NHS) in the UK. I felt as though I had just been granted permission and justification to bring aspects of spirituality into sessions in a more open way and EMDR was providing the bridge to unite these two worlds.

EMDR and I seemed to develop a natural bond from the start; like putting on a glove that fits snugly and feels familiar, warm and safe. One of the trainers, John Spector, observed the passion and enthusiasm in me, which gave me the strength and motivation to progress with my practitioner accreditation as soon as possible. Within a short period of time, I took on a newly created role within the service where I was working, as trauma lead for a Child and Adolescent Mental Health Service (CAMHS). After some trepidation I settled into this role quickly, offering peer supervision and looking at ways to introduce a trauma pathway for clients. Sadly, the service (and possibly many similar services in the country) was not quite ready for trauma pathways and despite my best attempts, many of my projects were halted. By this stage my soul, unbeknown to me, had another plan. It is fair to say that at this point I did feel the universe gave me a huge push; leaving a relatively 'stable' environment with a pension, holiday entitlement and other perks, I took a significant leap of faith and found myself setting up as an independent clinician. The idea would have been daunting a few years earlier, as my ego clung to the small perks of apparent safety, but I found myself on my own and having to trust and surrender to the bigger picture.

I have never looked back; my soul clearly knew what it was doing and the clients appeared with minimal effort. I started to appreciate that I could now work in a much more authentic, clinical way, unconstrained by bureaucracy and politics. With time my spirituality blended into my work seamlessly. My EMDR journey continued as I joined the EMDR UK Child & Adolescent Committee in 2016 and before long I found myself acting in the role of Chair, which I continued for four years. This opened up horizons and opportunities to connect and offer trainings with some special souls. However, it wasn't until 2019 that my soul planted the idea of setting up the UK's Special Interest Group (SIG) in EMDR & Spirituality and it was here that I felt I had really landed home. I had just completed my first book introducing spirituality into clinical practice using Heart Led Psychotherapy (HLP; Dent, 2020) and the SIG offered a safe environment in which to share such ideas with like-minded colleagues.

My own spiritual journey

Alongside my clinical work, I would consider the most important aspect of working spiritually with clients is to embrace one's own spiritual journey. Whilst I had always held a strong faith system, I had little confidence and trust in myself or my abilities. Alternative therapies and healing are something I have naturally been drawn to and explored from a young age. However, I embarked on a major spiritual transition in 2016, the first seven years of which was intense and it was during this time that I developed HLP. HLP provides a spiritually informed working model; guiding individuals to become more heart led and authentic, sometimes taking huge leaps of faith to break out of familiar egoic patterns and beliefs that maintain distress and suffering. This spiritual healing phase of my life involved deep clearing, healing and integration of many, many soul blocks and restrictions from current and past lives and it's fair to say I frequented some very dark and uncomfortable places during the process.

I must also admit that during this spiritual transition, I naively dived into the spiritual world/community in my search to try and understand myself more fully and heal my underlying soul blocks and wounds. I was determined that I didn't want to keep coming back lifetime after lifetime going around the repetitive hamster wheel of traumatic cycles. Whilst I was actively seeking a healthier, more authentic version of myself, for several years I was still having encounters and connections that were traumatic but familiar. I was delving deeper into the onion, peeling back more and more layers, shedding relationships that no longer resonated and connecting with others that were facilitating my healing and learning. I hadn't recognised how trauma was so familiar to me and my nervous system and whilst it wasn't desirable, it was what I knew. There were times where I felt I was shedding almost everything from my life which was a frightening and lonely place to be.

I also hadn't appreciated how much ego there is within the spiritual community, just as there is outside of it. The availability and variety of different spiritual techniques and concepts is constantly on the increase and readily accessible, both online and in person, including information and ideas which promote the 'right way' to spiritually ascend or awaken; how to reach higher levels of awareness, operate at higher dimensions or frequencies, or finally individuals who believed that they have been 'given' activation codes to help you progress in your spiritual journey.

When I started embracing this part of my spiritual journey, I fell into the trap of believing what I was hearing and seeing. I was perhaps in a vulnerable place, making massive changes in my life and looking for support and guidance outside of me. I was aware at some level that what people said and how they behaved didn't always match up and observed a lack of authenticity, but I hadn't built up enough trust and self-belief to really challenge this. It was only through the process of having had some tough encounters, in tandem with undergoing enormous amounts of soul level healing, that I started to become more aware and accepting that what I was witnessing and experiencing wasn't always aligning with my heart, soul and authenticity. If I am honest, my soul usually gave me the signal at the beginning; that internal deep alarm, but I hadn't learned to trust this signal. At some level I believe I needed to have the experiences I did, to be able to fully recognise what was happening and to finally make more healthier heart led choices. I was choosing to walk the walk the hard way!

Nowadays, I am much more discerning about what I listen to and participate in. As time progressed, my soul increasingly showed me that I needed to keep coming back to within. I was being shown that none of us are lacking in any way; we all have what we need within ourselves. This is where we really find our own truth and authenticity and it is to be expected that this truth and authenticity may vary between individuals. Being authentic is possible for every single one of us, regardless of our backgrounds, and shouldn't be determined by affordability or the number of spiritual courses, retreats or trainings you have attended. I am not suggesting for one minute that we shouldn't access genuine support along the way because this is often required, but this is done in combination with and in balance with working on ourselves too.

This book

This book aims to find an approach that is suitable for anyone, regardless of their spiritual or religious beliefs, by providing a framework that is heart led; bridging science with spirituality, western traditions with eastern traditions. My perspective of this topic is informed by my own personal and spiritual journey as well as by my professional experience. My clinical experience has been in the NHS and private practise in the UK for 25 years, mostly with white European individuals across the age span but also with individuals from different socio-economic backgrounds, race, sexual orientation, gender and culture. I acknowledge that I do not have extensive experience of working with racialised and other marginalised groups.

The book will take you on a journey of how to embody spirituality into your EMDR clinical practice, with the first part providing an overview of transpersonal psychology, spirituality and working energetically within therapy. Please note that these are huge areas to cover and it is not within the remit of this book to go into detail about different spiritual or religious groups, organisations or practices. These can be explored elsewhere if interested. The second part of the book focuses on key areas of HLP, including the ego, mindfulness and benefits of working at a heart level, as well as how to teach your clients HLP. The third and final part focuses on incorporating spirituality into EMDR therapy; taking you through each of the eight phases, before finally addressing some other considerations and clinical areas, including EMDR supervision. Some of the content about working spiritually and Heart Led Psychotherapy (HLP) and all the figures and tables have been taken from my previous book, *Using Spirituality in Psychotherapy* published by Routledge in 2020 and reproduced here by permission of Taylor & Francis Group.

As you read this book, I am going to invite you to consider two main things: spiritual experiences cannot easily be proven in current times, so just because something hasn't happened to you or isn't your experience doesn't mean it doesn't happen to others. The word 'spirituality' in itself can be quite triggering and divisive for some. If you do feel triggered by anything, try to go within and explore what this may be highlighting for you; is there an inner wound that would benefit from healing? Please keep an open mind and heart and adopt a position of non-judgement and curiosity. Always connect in your heart and soul as you learn or hear about new information or experiences to find your own truth and don't adopt mine or others readily. Secondly, and as I often say to clients, colleagues and friends, if it resonates then enjoy, if not then leave behind.

Acknowledgements

Firstly, a huge sense of gratitude to Francine Shapiro for having the insight, courage and commitment to develop EMDR. EMDR has positively impacted so many individuals' lives over more than four decades and will continue to evolve and be such a powerful life changing intervention.

I want to thank the clients that I have worked with during my career. I could not have developed and applied HLP without your support and input. As I've discussed in this book, I do believe that we are all each other's teachers and mirrors, some stronger than others, but all here to support one another on our own individual journey. I am always struck by what an honour and privilege it is when clients feel safe enough to be vulnerable, trust and have the courage to open up to work through their difficulties with me. I hope that I never take this for granted and remain humble and always open to learning and growing. An especially big thank you to those clients who agreed to be case studies. Your personal stories are what brings the book to life.

Secondly, I would like to thank my publisher Susannah Frearson, whose enthusiasm from the start enabled me to swiftly transgress from a proposal about updating my previous book to proposing a book in its own right. It all happened within 48 hours and I was thrilled when we could get EMDR in the title and focus this book specifically on EMDR therapy. I finally realised this is what I had been working towards all the time and all the pieces of the jigsaw puzzle smoothly and seamlessly fell into place. Alongside this, thank you to Ian Barron, Sandi Richman and Irene Siegel for encouraging and supporting me with this project. I am also grateful to Beverly Coghlan who kindly made time early in the process to support me with sourcing various research articles. I am indebted to my lovely friend and colleague Amanda Wood for her permission to use her stunning painting as the front cover image; it represents such a special spiritual place of mine.

I entrusted the first draft of the book into the tender care of my special and blessed friend Nic Hartshorne. I knew you would be compassionate but also honest with me, and at times challenge and pull me up when needed to make sure the content evolved into an authentic version of my work. You have been such a dear support in my life over the past few years on the UK Special

Interest Group in EMDR and Spirituality, a rock to keep me grounded and give me strength. Sadly, another massive support, Julie Dorey, did not live to see this venture through, and she now shines as a beautiful star in the night sky; your dear sweet soul will remain forever in my heart and you are so missed.

To those that I have worked with over the years on various UK EMDR Association committees, thank you for your friendship, collaboration and guidance. An especially big sense of gratitude to Mike O'Connor and Ali Russell (aka Mumma and Pappa bear) who have held me through some dark times and always believed in me; you are more special to me than you could possibly know.

There are two key people in my life who have recently supported me through so much turbulence and always held a place of compassion, kindness and unconditional positive regard and love for me. The first is Vivien Rushmere. You are a great example of trusting in Divine timings. We first worked together in the same NHS Trust 22 years ago, but were in different physical locations, so our paths rarely crossed. However, I felt a deep connection and recognition with your soul from the beginning. It was when you contacted me five years ago, when you were setting yourself up as a private clinician, that we both had space in our lives to develop and deepen our friendship. I regard you as one of my angel wings. The other angel wing is my dear friend, supervisor and colleague, Alice Vine. You have been everything to me and I am so grateful for your friendship, support, belief, time and respect. You are an incredible soul, and I couldn't have written this book without you.

Thank you to those that have helped with versions of the editing and providing valuable feedback including Nicki Fayers, Michelle Sorrell, Rotem Brayer and Jamie Hacker Hughes. Your input has been gratefully received. A massive thank you to Irene Siegel for kindly agreeing to write a Foreword to this book; your expertise, knowledge, wisdom and support have been greatly appreciated throughout this process.

My friendships and relationships have evolved and changed during my journey, many have parted, some have remained and some have arrived anew. The ones I have in my life now are more authentic and heart felt and a joy to know and spend time with. They help keep me grounded and focused in the present moment. You know who you are, so thank you with deep gratitude for being you.

Lastly, to my biggest teachers and mirrors; my beautiful children Olivia and Sebastian. What a journey! You have taught me to completely surrender and trust in the unknown and often I have had to learn this the hard way. You are incredible souls and have so much potential; thank you from the bottom of my heart. May you stay safe, be well and embrace your amazing journeys with strength, courage and hope. I love you both dearly.

Foreword

Are you a therapist navigating the crossroads of conventional psychotherapy and the emerging fields of higher consciousness and spirituality? Or perhaps you're an individual seeking the right therapy to heal past trauma and awaken spiritually. If so, this book will be a valuable resource for you. *Using Spirituality in EMDR Therapy: The Heart Led Approach* presents a unique integration of Eye Movement Desensitization and Reprocessing (EMDR) therapy with spiritual awakening, offering a comprehensive guide to healing through both psychological and spiritual methods.

Alexandra Dent, a Clinical Psychologist, EMDR therapist, and consultant, guides readers through her innovative approach—blending EMDR with spiritual principles to foster heart-centered healing. Her book provides practical exercises and meditations designed to enhance mindfulness and elevate consciousness, paving the way for a deeper integration of spirituality within therapeutic practice.

The integration of spirituality and psychotherapy has a rich history that dates back to the early days of psychology when pioneers like Carl Jung explored the connection between the psyche and spiritual experience. Over the decades, the field has evolved, with a growing recognition of the importance of addressing both the mind and the spirit in the healing process. Approaches such as transpersonal psychology and humanistic psychology have paved the way for a more holistic view of mental health, where spiritual growth is seen as a vital component of well-being. EMDR therapy, with its innovative techniques for processing trauma, fits naturally into this trend by offering a structured yet flexible framework that can incorporate spiritual elements. By addressing trauma not just as a psychological event but as a profound spiritual experience, EMDR allows for a deeper, more comprehensive healing journey that resonates with the soul's quest for wholeness.

As a fellow EMDR therapist, consultant, author, and speaker, I, Irene Siegel, have dedicated my work to merging transpersonal approaches with EMDR therapy, drawing from the teachings of ancient wisdom traditions. I am particularly drawn to Dent's work because it mirrors my own journey in the United States, while she leads a parallel path in the United Kingdom. We both chair EMDR Special Interest Groups focusing on spirituality, and our serendipitous collaboration has been mutually enriching.

Dent's unique 'Heart Led Approach' evolves into a model she terms 'Heart Led Psychotherapy' (HLP). This approach helps clients distinguish between the ego's perceptions and the soul's awareness, guiding them from external identification to the emergence of their authentic self. For EMDR therapists seeking a deeply relational approach within a spiritual context while maintaining the integrity of EMDR protocols, this book offers profound insights.

Throughout the eight phases of EMDR therapy, Dent provides a road map to integrate the HLP as part of a BioPsychoSocioSpiritual framework. Her compassionate, heart-to-heart method encourages clients to use mindfulness and meditation during the silent spaces of processing, creating internal resources for self-soothing and regulation. This process supports clients in exploring deeper levels of consciousness, including past life experiences, soul connections, and cosmic awareness, thereby redefining trauma beyond the cognitive memory of the present lifetime. Identifying the gifts within the trauma, and the life lessons that it brings within the soul's journey give positive meaning to experiences that allow the client to go beyond healing creating a future template driven by spiritual awakening.

As we enter an age of awakening—what the Mayans refer to as the Golden Age—people are increasingly becoming aware of their interconnectedness with all living things. This shift in consciousness necessitates a corresponding evolution in psychological practice. Dent's work provides a pioneering transpersonal model of psychotherapy that includes considerations of past lives and soul awareness, offering a bridge to new therapeutic paradigms.

Whether you are an experienced EMDR therapist, a professional interested in exploring EMDR, or an individual seeking the right therapeutic path, there is something invaluable in this book for you. I highly recommend it. *Enjoy your journey into a transpersonal model of EMDR through a heart led approach!*

Best regards,

Irene R. Siegel, Ph.D., LCSW

A spiritual perspective into psychotherapy

Chapter I

Transpersonal psychology and EMDR

'Do not feel lonely, the entire universe is within you.'

Rumi

This chapter focuses on a transpersonal approach with psychotherapy including EMDR therapy. Whilst it is beyond the scope of this book to provide too much detail or depth into what could be considered a very complex area, an overview and background to the key founders and core concepts of transpersonal psychotherapy is provided. Different forms that the process of spiritual awakening can take are then discussed, which may also occur as a result of experiencing trauma. How transpersonal ideas have been incorporated into EMDR over the past 20 years is then discussed along with the few transpersonal protocols that have been developed during this time. Lastly, the idea of working therapeutically within the quantum field is explored including how this can be achieved within EMDR therapy.

Transpersonal psychology

Transpersonal psychology is a branch or approach within psychology that explores and understands human experiences and psychological distress from a spiritual, transcendent and transformational aspect. It literally means 'beyond the person.' It attempts to integrate traditional psychological ideas with more spiritual and mystical experiences, including religious and philosophical traditions. It is the bridging together of Eastern and Western practices, science and spirituality, the fostering of personal and collective transformation and a move away from a dualistic perspective towards nondualism in order to reach one's highest potential. Other concepts considered significant within transpersonal psychology include a connection with nature, holistic healing, experiences from psychedelic therapy, spiritual crisis and emergence.

Transpersonal psychology evolved in the 1960s and 1970s and is considered the Fourth Force in Psychology, where psychology has moved from a behavioural, to a psychoanalytical, to a humanistic, and finally, a transpersonal

DOI: 10.4324/9781003509646-2

approach. William James, considered by many to be the father of American psychology, had a significant influence on the foundation of transpersonal psychology. His work included subjective experiences of individuals in religious or mystical states, stream of consciousness and pluralism, as well as encouraging an open and pragmatic approach in philosophy. James provided the groundwork for many modern psychological theories and practices.

Carl Jung's work has also been very influential in the development of transpersonal psychology. His spiritual training with Indian Hindu gurus and his own personal experiences, often through dream analysis, led him to write about the collective unconscious and archetypes. Jung (1959a) introduced the concept of collective unconsciousness to describe the part of the unconscious mind shared by all humans, which contains inherited experiences of all cultures, ages and archetypes, including those where there is no intellectual knowledge. An archetype refers to a universal symbol, pattern or intense meaning state, that appears across cultures and throughout history and can trigger deep and sometimes unconscious responses in an individual. Examples of archetypes include the hero, rescuer, martyr, trickster, mother, bully, caregiver or lover. An archetype is permanent; an essence or universal principle that helps give rise to meaning in the world and can hold a 'numinous' quality that may be divine, spiritual or religious. Numinous experiences may be felt with different levels of intensity sometimes going beyond ordinary states of comprehension, have intense powerful positive emotions and be experienced in a profound way. Archetypal crisis can occur when someone has a numinous experience and then struggles to integrate this back into their present reality.

Jung's four main archetypes included the persona, shadow, anima/animus and the self. The 'Self' is an archetype which signified the unity of the conscious with the unconscious to represent the psyche as a whole. Whilst Jung believed that the Self transcends the ego, it also includes the ego as one of its components. When the ego, or conscious identity, is in dialogue with the Self, it enables individuals to align their conscious values with the deeper wisdom of the unconscious. He used the term 'individuation' to describe the process of integrating unconscious material into the consciousness to recognise one's own unique identity and facilitate greater self-awareness, wholeness and a more meaningful life. Jung described the 'Shadow' archetype as the dark side of the Self. He postulated that the Shadow usually represents the part of ourselves we do not like, the part we try and mask, hide and avoid within ourselves and the world around us. Jung considered that learning to connect with one's Shadow was an essential part of spiritual healing. An authentic existence could be achieved through practising self-awareness, integrating one's Shadow, aligning with the Self, embracing one's unique qualities and using creative expression such as writing, music and art.

Another influential and key contributor in the 1960s to the growth of the transpersonal psychology movement was Joseph Campbell, a world-famous writer and mythologist, who was influenced by Jung's work and archetypes. In his most famous work, the 'Hero's Journey' which can be found in his volume, *The Hero with a Thousand Faces* (Campbell, 2012), he describes how a protagonist ventures out on an unforeseen quest to face various mysterious challenges and encounters. During this experience the protagonist gains insights and returns home transformed. This powerful narrative framework is a story that resonates with many individuals on a spiritual journey because it captures universal human experiences of growth and transformation by overcoming adversity. It involves separating oneself from a sense of comfort and familiarity to explore the unknown, increasing one's awareness and undertaking various challenges (rather than trying to avoid or bypass) to integrate the learning and so return transformed.

Early key therapists involved in the transpersonal psychology movement also include Assagioli (founder of Psychosynthesis), Maslow (co-founding Humanistic Psychology) and Grof (founder of holotropic breathwork). Maslow & Grof explored a transpersonal dimension to access altered states of consciousness that transcend the ego, time, space and empirical reality, so that one can connect with a divine force. Grof conducted a great deal of research with psychedelics in the 1960s and 1970s, in particular with lysergic acid diethylamide (LSD), exploring the benefits of psychedelic-assisted psychotherapy not only for treating various mental health conditions, but also as a means to facilitate spiritual experiences and personal transformation. He developed the concept of the Basic Perinatal Matrix which proposed that birth-related trauma was a significant contributor to emotional difficulties later on in life. He believed that some individuals were able to access expanded or altered states of consciousness (through the use of psychedelics or holotropic breathwork) to connect with new perspectives when re-experiencing and healing emotional and psychological difficulties related to their birth. Grof & Grof (2010) proposed that spiritual experiences can occur in two distinct ways. The first, known as 'the immanent Divine' explains how an individual does not perceive any boundaries between themselves and the world around them (including with others, animals, nature and inanimate objects). They viewed everything as part of a unified field of cosmic creative energy and any perceived boundaries are unreal or illusory; they are at one with all that is and everything around them is an expression of themselves. The second way, known as 'the transcendental Divine' involves transcending beyond the everyday world and state of consciousness to connect with archetypal beings and realms. Grof and Grof believed it is possible to transcend linear time to experience and connect with ancestors, racial and karmic patterns and phylogenetic sequences as well as aspects of the collective unconscious.

Process of spiritual awakening

Spiritual awakening is a very personal and transformative experience that can manifest in a variety of different ways, depending on one's own beliefs, cultural background and journey. It can include a sudden awakening where often a significant life event or spiritual experience results in a profound shift in consciousness or awareness. For some it may be more gradual over time, connecting with various insights or changes in perspective with periods of growth, reflection and integration. Another form of spiritual awakening may occur as a result of the activation of Kundalini energy. This is an energy that is believed to reside at the base of the spine in Hindu and Yogic traditions and once activated, it moves up the energy centres (chakras) in the spine resulting in heightened awareness and a sense of connection and unity with the cosmos. Other forms of awakening include having a Near Death Experience (NDE), Dark Night of the Soul experience, awakening to a sense of oneness, purpose or presence in one's life, or having a spiritual crisis or emergency (a sudden and intense identity crisis, usually resulting from a spiritual experience where one's meaning system drastically changes).

White (1994) introduced the term 'Exceptional Human Experiences' (EHEs) to describe the various extraordinary experiences that individuals were reporting to have, which had the potential to be transformative during psychotherapy. This included psychic (telepathy, precognition, psychokinesis and clairvoyance), altered states of consciousness (occurring during meditation, trance or psychedelic experiences), NDE, out of body experiences (OBE), mystical experiences and encounters with apparitions or ghosts.

Various renowned spiritual leaders, such as Rumi and the Indian spiritual master Sathya Sai Baba, have described three stages in the awakening process:

- The first involves an awareness to presence (outside of oneself).
- The second stage is the journey with presence (within oneself).
- The last stage is the experience of the 'I am' presence (nondual awareness).

If we take, for example, learning to connect to a Divine Source; firstly a person will see the Divine outside of them, before moving to an awareness of the Divine within themselves and lastly a recognition that they are the Divine. In this process, a person is able to transcend the three-dimensional world they reside in.

Steve Taylor (2017) describes the spiritual journey as a form of awakening. In order to stay awake, one must first start leaving a state of sleep by keeping the eyes open and staying in the moment. Psychological distress and trauma have been shown to be one of the key triggers to a spontaneous awakening (Taylor & Egeto-Szabo, 2017; Taylor, 2019), where a person goes within in order to seek meaning from the experiences. A transpersonal approach to psychotherapy and healing encourages exploration of all aspects of life and the world and our existence within it, including 'who or what am I?' and 'what is the meaning of life?' and facilitates a client in the process of moving between the different stages of awakening. During the therapeutic relationship or resonance, the transpersonal therapist, working with an open heart and soul and connected with their true authentic self, does not view their client as being fundamentally different from themselves. This provides a space in which the client can begin to explore and discover their own authenticity and inner presence within a peaceful, safe and contained setting. Krystal et al. (2002) suggest that a transpersonal approach supports clients in realising that it is their thoughts that cause distress. By learning to live a more mindful, present life and releasing the need to be either caught in the past, or concerned about the future, clients can experience less suffering and learn to let go of attachments to things or people that are keeping them stuck. A transpersonal psychotherapist is able to see the wholeness and completeness within their client, even when the client is unable to recognise this at first themselves. Walsh & Vaughan (1993, p. 203) described transpersonal psychology as: 'experiences in which the sense of identity or self extends beyond (trans) the individual or personal to encompass wider aspects of humankind, life, psyche or cosmos.' A more detailed interpretation is provided by Caplan (2009, p. 231) who proposed:

> Transpersonal psychologists attempt to integrate timeless wisdom and modern Western psychology and translate spiritual principles into scientifically grounded, contemporary language. Transpersonal psychology addresses the full spectrum of human psychospiritual development – from our deepest wounds and needs, to the existential crisis of human being, to the most transcendent capacities of our consciousness.

Whilst Watts (2018) questioned whether the term transpersonal actually relates to something beyond the individual, Siegel (2018) advocated that the aim is to help individuals go beyond the healing of their trauma through an awakening process so that they can achieve their highest potential.

What is EMDR?

Eye Movement Desensitisation and Reprocessing (EMDR) is a powerful trauma therapy originally developed by Francine Shapiro in 1987. When a person experiences a trauma or significant life event, fragments of that memory (including image, thoughts, sensory experiences and emotions) are believed to be frozen in time and isolated in their own neural network, held in a dysfunctional, non-adaptive and state-specific form. This can prevent the brain from processing the memory. Connecting with an unprocessed traumatic memory, even long after the event has happened, can make a person feel as if they are still experiencing symptoms of the trauma. Although the exact mechanism is still unclear, EMDR uses an adaptive information processing (AIP) model to enable the fragments of the memory to connect to appropriate associations and be processed towards an adaptive and healthy resolution (Shapiro, 2018).

EMDR consists of eight distinguishable phases: history-taking, preparation, assessment, desensitisation, installation, body scan, closure and re-evaluation. The AIP system is activated during phase four, the desensitisation phase, using bilateral dual attention. This is when an individual is firstly asked to connect to the worst moment of a trauma and identify the:

- Image.
- Negative cognition (NC).
- Positive cognition (PC).
- Validity of the positive cognition (VOC) on a scale of 1 to 7, where 1 represents completely false and 7 represents completely true.
- Emotions.
- Subjective units of distress (SUDS) on a scale of 0 to 10 where 10 represents the worst possible and 0 represents no disturbance.
- Body location.

The therapist then uses bilateral stimulation (BLS) using eye movements, sound or tapping to stimulate the brain from left to right, in sets, usually between 24 to 28 BLS per cycle. After each set, the client is asked to briefly describe what they noticed happen. This continues until all aspects of the memory have been processed to an adaptive resolution.

In phase five, the installation phase, the positive cognition is paired with the original memory and BLS is applied to enhance the validity of the positive belief until it is completely true (VOC is 7/7). It isn't always possible to complete the processing of a distressing memory during one session, especially if the memory was very traumatic. To make sure that the client leaves the sessions in a positive frame of mind, they are asked to connect to one of the resources they have learnt in the preparation phase, typically their 'safe/calm place' (Shapiro, 2018). Alternatively, they can be asked 'what is the most important or meaningful thing that has come out of the work we did today?' Ideally, the therapist looks for a self-referencing positive statement that can be installed using slow BLS, allowing the client to leave the session in a calm and resourced state.

EMDR was originally developed for clients with Post Traumatic Stress Disorder (PTSD) for which there is now a wealth of literature, including randomised control trials, which illustrate the effectiveness of EMDR in treating this disorder. Additionally, its effectiveness for healing trauma is also recognised by the World Health Organization (2013). EMDR has also been researched and demonstrated to be an effective therapy for many different psychological difficulties including: anxiety, depression, obsessive compulsive disorder, psychosis and much more. It can also be used with young children where developmental modifications are applied (e.g. Tinker & Wilson, 1999; Lovett, 2015). EMDR is therefore an effective therapy to treat unprocessed memories that underlie trauma or significant life events.

EMDR and Transpersonal Psychology

A transpersonal EMDR therapist is not only committed to their own spiritual journey and healing but also recognises the potential for multi-dimensional healing and spiritual awakening in their clients, holding an awareness of present reality with a connection to a greater cosmic whole.

Several different authors have recognised how a spiritual component can be applied when using EMDR, for example, Parnell (1996, 2008); Krystal et al. (2002), R. Shapiro (2009), Dobo (2015, 2023); Hacker Hughes (2017); Siegel (2017, 2018), and Dent (2020, 2021). Similarities between EDMR and Vipassana meditation was reported by Parnell (1996) particularly in relation to dual attention or awareness, as well as encouraging the client to notice whatever arises during the process without judgement. Parnell (1996) and others (as referenced above) also discussed how EMDR processing and meditation facilitated clients in reaching a place of compassion and inner truth, sometimes leading to a new sense of inner spiritual connection and the ability to go beyond their egos to connect with transcendent or cosmic experiences. This is consistent with my clinical observations in my own EMDR clinical practice. Parnell (2008) wrote about different types of spiritual resources that can be used with EMDR clients, including spiritual figures, connecting with a higher power, the essential spiritual self, wise beings and spiritual experiences and teachings (which are discussed further in Chapter 10). Robin Shapiro (2009) devoted a chapter in her book *EMDR Solutions II* to working with religious and spiritually attuned clients based on her experience as a pastoral psychotherapist, theologian, clergyperson and clinician. She described adopting a 'fourth ear' to listen out for any information from the client that might have a religious or spiritual experience or context that could be used either as a positive resource or identified as a trauma that might be in conflict with their faith or tradition.

Krystal et al. (2002) developed a transpersonal EMDR protocol that can be used when all previous traumas or issues have been processed and the client is interested in exploring more fundamental questions about who they are and their purpose in life. The main focus of this protocol is to reduce external distractions and noise of the mind, emotions and sensations to facilitate a deeper inner connection and sense of contentment. The protocol is broken down into four key phases as follows:

- In the first phase, clients are asked to review their life whilst long sets of bilateral stimulation (BLS) are administered. This may provide insight into the various learning opportunities and lessons that their current life has provided so far. During this phase, the next step is to facilitate the client to experience a state of contentment using various exercises or techniques including prayer or meditation.
- The second phase of the protocol, equivalent to the EMDR assessment phase of the standard protocol, establishes a contentment baseline by

releasing any distractions that are stopping the client from being fully present. In this phase clients are asked to 'quiet down' over a period of 10 to 15 minutes before rating the level of quietness or contentment achieved ('light' meaning they are very distracted, 'medium' or 'deep' meaning they are not distracted at all). Targets are then identified for any distractions that are taking the person away from a sense of contentment as previously established during the baseline measure and these are scored using a level of distraction (LOD) scale, where 10 equates to very distracting and 0 is not at all distracting.

- During the third phase (the processing phase), clients are invited to connect with each target that was identified previously as distracting and BLS is applied. When all targets have reduced their LOD to 0/10 then the client is asked to reconnect with their baseline contentment for a further 10 to 20 minutes. Any additional distractions that emerge during the processing can be identified and targeted using the same procedure. The idea is that with practice, clients become more able to find contentment by adopting self-awareness and the role of observer to release distractions.
- The final phase encourages clients to ground themselves and to document any new distractions in between sessions.

Whilst I do not have any personal experience of using such a protocol, it does sound very similar to assisting clients in the process of adopting a more mindful, present way of living.

Dobo (2015) noticed a parallel between his clinical work with EMDR clients and Jung's individuation process. Dobo believed that EMDR could activate the soul to accelerate the individuation process, facilitating an opportunity to continually grow and evolve throughout one's lifetime. He also aligned the EMDR journey with the six-stage Christian Passion experience from death to rebirth. Dobo (2015) provided a map of the soul (or map of the human psyche) which he used with clients to illustrate the journey. To summarise:

- Stage one, Gethsemane, represents avoidance.
- Stage two, surrender to God's will, represents the ability to surrender.
- Stage three, crucifixion, represents dismantling of the old self.
- Stage four, three days in the tomb, represents chaos/loss of identity and a time of creative introversion which is critical for transformation to occur.
- Stage five, resurrection, represents rebirth process.
- Stage six, ascension, represents integrating the new self.

Dobo emphasised that the journey is not often linear or logical and one can be in more than one stage at any given time. He developed this further to also integrate Jungian psychology and the 12 stages of Campbell's monomyth, the Hero's Journey, into his EMDR therapy (Dobo, 2023), providing a therapeutic map that represents the client's heroic journey to their authentic self.

Although not exclusively for EMDR trained therapists, Botkins (2000) developed the Induced After Death Communication (IADC) protocol to use with EMDR clients, in which the core goal was to reduce the intense sadness and emotional distress associated with grief and loss. This was generally achieved within two EMDR sessions each of approximately 90 minutes duration utilising BLS. Whilst saying that ADC isn't actually induced, Botkins suggested that it worked by supporting clients into a state of mind where ADC had more likelihood of occurring. He found that directly targeting and processing the feelings of loss facilitated a level of acceptance and helped diminish feelings of anger and guilt. Clients were asked to think about where they believed their deceased friend or loved one was right now, or 'hold the thought' of the deceased person and then BLS would be applied. If there was no spontaneous ADC, then the client was invited to imagine where the deceased person was now and what they would say to them. Elsaesser et al. (2020) reported that whilst religious beliefs only increased slightly after an ADC, spirituality was significantly heightened by the ADC experiences.

On 28 January 2024, Annabel McGoldrick presented a workshop to the UK's Special Interest Group in EMDR and Spirituality, discussing a protocol that she developed called 'Dialogue with Death.' This protocol assists therapists in supporting clients to have conversations with deceased loved ones. The therapist can assist the client to invite the deceased loved one's essence, soul or spirit into the session, perhaps asking them to take a seat on a comfortable chair in the room. ADC can take the form of various senses including visual, auditory, tactile or olfactory, and if no spontaneous ADC occurs, the therapist may ask: 'If you would like to say one thing to your deceased loved one what would that be?'

Over the past decade there has been a growing interest in exploring how to integrate spiritual healing practices within EMDR therapy to facilitate multi-dimensional healing. I am sure this will continue to deepen and expand with time as more and more therapists connect or reconnect with their own healing innate abilities. A key contributor in the field of EMDR is Irene Siegel, an EMDR consultant and shamanic practitioner based in America who is a frequent presenter, teacher, supervisor and writer (Siegel, 2013, 2017, 2018, 2019). Shamans are considered by some to be the caretakers of the earth and believe that trauma is held vibrationally within the human energy field, whether it is from a current lifetime or an ancestral one. Shamans learn to move between non-ordinary reality and the ordinary world using processes such as mindfulness and meditation to help clear old patterns and beliefs, so that the individual can find peace and harmony. In her publications since 2017, Siegel has illustrated in some detail how this ancient form of healing is interwoven into her EMDR sessions by establishing a shared energy field between herself and clients, which is further deepened during the silent moments during BLS. She often uses sound or tactile BLS which enables clients to close their eyes (if clinically safe and appropriate) to facilitate potential movement into altered states of awareness during processing. Shamans also believe that when a person experiences trauma, a part of their soul can be lost and Siegel has reported that using shamanic healing techniques during EMDR can facilitate soul retrieval (2019). She described how clients working with transpersonal EMDR therapists could experience cosmic and EHEs during EMDR processing, including healing light, connecting with spiritual guides, or facilitators to enable multi-dimensional transpersonal healing of traumas. Siegel found that when experienced transpersonal EMDR therapists incorporated spiritual practice into their clinical work, a positive outcome was observed.

Sufism is a mystical and contemplative dimension of Islam which emphasises the direct personal experience of the divine. It has a rich array of spiritual practices such as dhikr (repeating divine names or phrases to remember God), meditation, contemplation and various devotional acts aimed at purifying the heart, attaining spiritual enlightenment and attaining union with the Divine. Abdul-Hamid & Hacker Hughes (2015) suggested that using certain religious and spiritual practises that have ritualistic movements such as Sufi dhikr, may provide a form of BLS and that these could be incorporated into EMDR to facilitate processing and make it more appealing and agreeable to a wider cultural population.

There is currently an increasing amount of interest in integrating the Internal Family Systems (IFS) model, developed by Richard Schwartz in the 1980s, into EMDR therapy. The model identifies a core or true Self, that can be found within everyone and has its own wisdom to heal all internal and external relationships. O'Malley (2018) developed sensorimotor-focused EMDR (SF-EMDR), integrating many spiritual concepts to provide a holistic and multi-dimensional way to heal clients. He suggested that SF-EMDR supports clients towards the 'path of the heart,' describing how his approach integrates information from the gut-brain and head-brain to achieve resonance at the level of the heart-brain.

Parnell (2008) made reference to life lessons that can be realised through life experiences although at the time of writing, found that they often remain unintegrated. I developed Heart Led Psychotherapy (HLP) as part of a BioPsychoSocioSpiritual approach to treating trauma (Dent, 2020) which is explained in more detail in subsequent chapters. HLP can be incorporated into EMDR therapy and enables life lessons to be understood and integrated using a transpersonal approach to clinical practice. Since publishing this work, I have also reconnected with the ancient healing of Light Language (a form of divine channelling energy and healing which is discussed in more detail in Chapter 8). I have presented at various workshops and conferences over the past few years on using Light Language in psychotherapy, including EMDR therapy, and examples of this will be illustrated throughout the book.

Working within the quantum field

The theoretical physicist, David Bohm (1917–1992) made significant contributions to the understanding of quantum mechanics and quantum theory when considering fundamental questions about the nature of reality, consciousness and human existence and viewed the universe as a complex, infinite, multi-dimensional, multi-layered thought form. Some key areas of his work include the idea of implicate and explicate orders to explain the relationship between the observable and tangible reality that we encounter in everyday experiences (the explicate order) and the deeper underlying reality (the implicate order). He proposed that the implicate order contained the potential for all things which unfolds into the explicate order as perceived reality. His idea of the 'holomovement' suggested that the universe is in a constant state of flux and interconnectedness, where every part of existence is dynamically related to every other part transcending the notions of space and time.

In his book *Becoming Supernatural*, Joe Dispenza (2017) discusses how the quantum field is beyond time, space and ego and believed to reside in the 5th dimension (5D), whereas we in physical form currently reside in the 3rd dimension (3D). He suggests that it is only possible to enter the quantum field through awareness or consciousness and one has to release all connections and attachments with the 3D world, moving from being 'somebody' to 'nobody.' The quantum field cannot be experienced through our senses; it is only blackness and is also referred to as the 'zero point' field. Learning to live a mindful life and be in the present moment enables one to enter the quantum field and access all the infinite information, possibilities, spaces, dimensions, realms, frequencies, energy and knowledge available. Connecting and pairing the feeling of elevated emotions with what one desires (intention) for the future and imagining feeling them in the present moment, not only changes the gene expression and light field of an individual, but enables them to live in the future-present reality and attract new experiences that match and manifest this energy. Thus, the energy expressed in one's energetic field is learning to move away from the familiarity of trauma and suffering, to the unfamiliar of manifesting a more positive healthier outcome, which over time becomes the new familiar.

O'Malley (2024) incorporated ideas and research findings from quantum physics and introduced the term 'Quantum EMDR' or QEMDR, suggesting that it can be used to facilitate a broadening of the client's window of tolerance, especially in the dissociative client, thus enabling the reprocessing of traumatic material. O'Malley explored in depth what he proposed is the science behind what happens during QEMDR, including the neurophysiology as well as cognitive, emotional and sensorimotor mechanisms. He described using a machine (including headphones, buzzers or tactile units and lights) to apply BLS to the area in the body which is experiencing the greatest amount of distress, for example around the gut, throat and olfactory regions. He then suggested that offering intensive EMDR, which may last four to five hours in a day, enables the client to remain within their window of tolerance, although it can still take up to a week for such processed material to be integrated within the hippocampus. O'Malley worked with clients to find a suitable colour, shade and intensity of healing light and radiated this with his machine to the area of the body being worked on, in addition to the BLS. Ulanzi lights (a type of LED light) are used by the client to facilitate this process, altering the frequency and vibration as required. O'Malley also described activating the efferent and afferent connections with the head-brain, heart-brain and gut-brain connections during QEMDR. He discussed how anything is possible working with a client in the quantum field, including healing at a soul and intergenerational level, but his reference to the relational experience and spiritual resonance between client and therapist is limited.

Summary

- A transpersonal psychotherapy approach which evolved in the 1960s and 1970s takes into account spiritual, mystical, and transformative experiences that are 'beyond' the individual.
- Key contributors to the field of transpersonal psychotherapy explored how altered states of consciousness can transcend the ego, time and space and empirical reality to facilitate a connection with a divine force, adopting a non-dualistic approach to their work.
- Jung's incorporation of different archetypes, including the persona, self, shadow and anima/animus have been very influential in understanding aspects of the spiritual process.
- There are different forms that spiritual awakening can take, including a sudden awakening (perhaps through a significant life event or trauma) or more gradual over time, Kundalini awakening, NDE, spiritual crisis or emergency.
- Various EHEs can be experienced by clients which can facilitate transformation during therapy.
- A transpersonal approach to EMDR therapy has been explored for over 20 years supporting clients to go beyond their egos and connect with transcendent or cosmic experiences during processing.
- New ways of connecting to the quantum field as part of a spiritual journey and also within EMDR therapy are being explored.

Chapter 2

Working spiritually and energetically with clients

'You have to grow from the inside out. None can teach you, none can make you spiritual. There is no other teacher but your own soul.'

Swami Vivekananda

This chapter starts with an exploration of what is meant by the term 'spirituality,' including the concept of a soul, and how this can be embraced in different belief systems. Guidance is then provided on how to explore one's own spirituality and various questions are suggested to assist in this process. The benefits of working spiritually with clients are discussed, which includes accessing additional, positive resources that can be utilised within EMDR therapy. What to do if you or your client isn't spiritual is also covered. The next section of the chapter focuses on introducing the idea of working energetically with clients, which is an additional or alternative way of exploring aspects of spirituality, especially for those clients who are new to this area. This includes understanding ourselves as electromagnetic beings that vibrate at different energetic frequencies which change depending on the emotions we connect with at any given time. How a therapist can intentionally prepare themselves for working spiritually or energetically before, during, and after sessions as well as within the clinical space is detailed.

What is spirituality?

If you have been drawn to read this book, you probably have some level of curiosity about spirituality and may already be integrating a spiritual or transpersonal perspective in your therapy. Over the years, I have witnessed and appreciated the value of incorporating spirituality into my own clinical work as well as my personal life. Spirituality encompasses qualities such as compassion, bliss, joy and unconditional love, even during very challenging or traumatic times. Not only does it provide additional access to utilise positive resources for an individual, but it can, potentially, facilitate transformative multi-dimensional level healing. People have reported different ways to connect with their own personal spiritual faith, for example, through meditation,

DOI: 10.4324/9781003509646-3

faith, prayer, healing, our environment and nature, music, poetry and literature, art, people and relationships.

The World Health Organization recognised spirituality as an important component of mental health at their 37th Assembly in 1984 and on quality of life in 2006 (WHOQOL SRPB, 2006). In 1994, the category of 'Religious or Spiritual Problem' was introduced into the *Diagnostic and Statistical Manual of Mental Disorders* (DSM-4) to refer to religious or spiritual problems as non-pathological problems that resulted in distress, such as loss of faith, converting to a new faith, or questioning of spiritual values (American Psychiatric Association, 1994) . In 2013, the Royal College of Psychiatrists produced recommendations for psychiatrists on spirituality and religion. There are also ever-increasing formations of specialist interest groups and committees for clinicians in the area of spirituality and transpersonal psychology including professions such as psychiatry, psychology and counselling as well as those clinicians who are members of different therapeutic modalities, including EMDR.

There are various views and opinions on what is meant by the term 'spirituality,' which can make it extremely difficult to find a unanimous agreement on a definition. In the *Oxford English Dictionary*, spirituality is defined as: 'The quality of being concerned with the human spirit or soul as opposed to material or physical things.' The French idealist philosopher, Jesuit priest and palaeontologist Pierre Teilhard de Chardin (1975), wrote: 'we are not human beings having spiritual experiences, we are spiritual beings having human experiences.'

Daniel Sulmasy, a medical doctor and philosopher, encourages spirituality to be all embracing and inclusive, open to the idea that there is something beyond the physical, cognitive and emotional experiences in this present situation and lifetime without segregating any particular religious beliefs, referring to spirituality as:

> an individual's or a group's relationship with the transcendent, however that may be construed. Spirituality is about the search for transcendent meaning. Most people express their spirituality in religious practice. Others express their spirituality exclusively in their relationship with nature, music, the arts, or a set of philosophical beliefs or relationships with friends and family.
>
> (Sulmasy, 2002, p. 25)

In Buddhism, this is sometimes referred to as a consciousness. Others refer to this as God, Buddha, Mohammed, Spirit, Allah, Cosmic Christ, Tao, etc. The Brahmins refer to Brahma, a Hindu god that is deemed 'the creator' and associated with knowledge, creation and the Vedas. In other words, it is the Divine spark residing deep within all of us (Atman) and not the body/ego that is synonymous to the Brahma. Richard Bucke, a Canadian psychiatrist of the 19th century, described cosmic consciousness as representing a higher state of awareness or enlightenment, in which an individual experiences a deep sense of connection and unity with the universe and a greater awareness of how all things are interconnected. This is a state that, once achieved, is characterised by feelings of bliss, insight and a level of understanding that extends beyond human experience. In their work using holotropic breathwork, Grof & Grof (2010) introduced the term 'COEX,' that is, systems of condensed experiences, to describe the 'many layers of unconscious material that share similar emotions or physical sensations; the contributions to a COEX system come from different layers of the psyche' (p. 15). They suggested that traumatic memories from infancy, childhood and adult life form the superficial layers. The next layers are connected to emotions and physical sensations of the birth process, and the deepest layers of all are connected to transpersonal aspects of the psyche, including past lives, and various collective archetypes throughout time. The character, number and intensity of the COEX will vary from one person to another; it can be positive or negative and when triggered, can generate underlying emotions or physical sensations. This appears to be synonymous with identifying touchstone events/memories during the floatback technique of the EMDR process, where either a current memory or traumatic memory being explored has previous themes that hold a similar emotion, belief or physical sensation. Holotropic breathwork therapy though, has to date, been more open and embracing of the possibility of connecting with the divine and transpersonal experiences, including ancestral and collective archetypes.

Irene Siegel (2017) referred to a divine energy, or divine cosmic consciousness, which can be integrated with energy from the earth and the divine essence or souls within individuals. In reference to spirituality, I believe in a Divine Source that is the true source or energy of infinite, unconditional love. I believe that we, and everything around us, is an expression of the Divine. When our soul or our divine essence aligns with and embraces the Divine Source, we have the potential to reach a place of bliss or Dharma. There are many ancient and Indian religious meanings of Dharma and no single-word translation exists. Wayne Dyer publicly spoke and wrote extensively about Dharma as being where everything in life has a purpose. He referred to Dharma as what you live by, an inner calling within one's heart which becomes clear when you truly align yourself with the Divine Source (Dyer, 2013). Dyer suggested that this is when you start living your soul Dharma, where all aspects of your life are in alignment with your spiritual beliefs and there is no separation or segregation. It is certainly not an easy or smooth process to live and breathe one's authentic truth throughout the day unmasked.

The soul

Spirituality can, but doesn't have to, believe in the presence of a soul, although I, personally, do believe in this. Again, like spirituality, it is difficult to scientifically prove or find a universally accepted definition of a soul.

However, there is an understanding within the many different religions and philosophical studies that a soul is an incorporeal essence of a living being.

In the 'Collected Works of The Mother' (1972, p. 247), the soul is defined as: 'The divine spark that dwells at the centre of each being; it is identical with its Divine Origin; it is the Divine in man.' In his description of soul-centred psychotherapy, Powell (2018, p. 73) refers to the soul as 'the manifestation of spirit through form,' suggesting that everything has a soul, but that humans are more advanced to include self-consciousness or *awareness of awareness.*' Tomlinson (2012) refers to the soul as a pure spirit energy, which holds all of the memories and experiences from each incarnation. For me, the soul is an immortal, invisible energy, the divine within us that originated from the Divine Source of unconditional love. I believe the soul is connected to our higher selves and carries our infinite memories, experiences and knowledge.

If you would like to explore more about a soul's journey then I would recommend *Journey of Souls* (Newton, 2011) and subsequent publications by the same author. Like Newton, I see myself first and foremost as a soul. In essence, I believe I am a soul that resides in a physical body that has emotions, sensations and beliefs. In this lifetime I happen to be a white female, but that doesn't mean that I have always been incarnated as a white person or a female. I believe my soul holds all the information and memories of my past lives as well as challenges and traumas that I have experienced. Believing in a soul, or the concept of reincarnation however, is not essential nor is it a prerequisite for working spiritually with individuals.

Being open to everything

I do not define myself as belonging to a particular religion or group. I have certainly experimented throughout my life in the search of finding a group or organisation that fits with my belief system. I was bought up in the Catholic faith and whilst this presented much confusion, it continued to be a big part of my life until I went to university. As my spirituality widened and I questioned some Catholic viewpoints, I tried other religions and spiritualist and meditation groups. I do believe that there can be a great deal of comfort and support in belonging to a particular church, religion or spiritual group, especially in time of need or distress. However, despite this, I have recently found peace in accepting that there isn't one group or organisation that encapsulates my spiritual understanding; and perhaps this allows me to remain open to the variety of beliefs held by different individuals. I have also noticed that I have had deep, spiritual experiences not only through meditation but also through contact with certain individuals, nature, places and activities, for example, dancing, gardening, mantras and yoga.

I am open to belief in God, Jesus, Angels and Archangels, Buddha, all of the Ascended Masters (spiritually enlightened beings who underwent spiritual transformations during their incarnations as humans) who have gone before us, as well as many other belief systems. Therefore, if I am working with someone who believes in God, I am comfortable utilising their own beliefs in the work we do, if appropriate. The same applies to someone who may be Muslim or Buddhist or aligned with other faiths. As long as I am open to working with their belief system and hold on to the basic principles of acting in a loving, compassionate manner, I can work with whatever anyone brings. This doesn't preclude me from working with someone who has no spiritual belief system, as I don't see it as my role to try and convert individuals to any point of view. We are all permitted our own beliefs and I am highly respectful of this. I have to hold on to the position of being accepting and open and, when appropriate, curious in gaining an understanding a client's spirituality and beliefs without judgement or criticism. I always try to work with what is true to them.

Exploring spirituality within yourself

If you are interested in using a spiritual approach with your clients, it is important for you to be open to the concept of spirituality and be comfortable in your own beliefs without feeling the need to impose them onto anyone else. If you are new to the topic of spirituality and interested in discovering how to live a more spiritual life, I would highly recommend Wayne Dyer's film *The Shift*. It portrays how to live a more authentic life and how opportunities can present themselves to open up to this concept. It would also be an appropriate recommendation to your clients. If you are keen to embrace your own spiritual journey and authentic truth, it is important that you are prepared to engage with various ongoing daily practices that assist you in this process. With time, you will learn to adopt a transpersonal approach in all areas of your life; there is no separation. Working on the basis that you may only be able to take your clients as far as you are prepared to venture, then the more inner work you do, the more potential there is for you to support your clients in reaching their true potential. The clients who find their way to you will reflect back where you are on your spiritual journey and you will notice that as you deepen your own spirituality, you will be working with more clients who are open to or are keen to embrace and deepen a spiritual journey themselves.

A transpersonal therapist is able to provide a safe, containing, energetic space and opportunity for clients to explore healing in a multi-dimensional way. As your own spiritual awareness increases, so will your ability to identify signs or opportunities with clients that allow the topic of spirituality to open up. Practising mindfulness will strengthen your awareness within clinical work (this is discussed in Chapter 5). Mindfulness practice has been reported to increase a sense of trust and closeness with others (Kabat-Zinn, 1994). Daniel Siegel (2010) suggested that engaging in mindfulness allows therapists to attune to and resonate with their clients. Therapists using mindfulness have been shown to bring these skills to their clinical work, which can strengthen the therapeutic relationship (Aggs & Bambling, 2010). Laszlo (2009) discussed a 'biofield,' which is described as a universal energy field that extends beyond the body, environment, time and space. Irene Siegel conducted a heuristic research study investigating the impact of spiritual resonance between therapists and clients in order to explore the energetic interaction that can occur. She described spiritual resonance as: 'Vibrational patterns of greater cosmic wholeness experienced through soul awareness; inclusive of all forms of resonances; not component based; and transmitted multi-directionally in the energy field between therapist, client, Divine Source, and Earth' (Siegel 2013, p. 49).

During the process of resonance, it is suggested that one moves beyond the egoic mind to access a higher presence, cosmic energy or divine force, which can be very transformative and healing when working with clients. As you move along your spiritual journey you may start noticing your intuition develop. This can occur in the form of physical sensations, a sense of knowing, inner hearing and seeing, sometimes referred to as clairvoyance (sight), claircognizance (knowledge), clairaudience (sound), clairalience (smell), clairsentience (feeling) or clairgustance (taste). These are all symptoms that I experience and they have been reported elsewhere (e.g., Braud & Anderson, 1998; Siegel, 2013).

Spiritual questions to explore within yourself

When you are working within a spiritual framework, you should aim to achieve cultural competency (which is also applied within all our clinical work). This is the ability to understand, appreciate, respect and interact with others from different cultures or belief systems to your own.

Below are some important questions to ask YOURSELF before starting such work with your clients. If you are used to meditating then you can use this process to discover your answers and notice how they make you feel. There are no right or wrong answers to any of these questions, just observe what is true to you at this given stage in your life journey. Try to explore these questions with an openness and acceptance and without judgement or criticism of yourself and others, adopting a level of self-enquiry and curiosity. It may be helpful to hold in mind certain key themes that may be unconsciously biasing your responses, including your social identity (sex, gender, race, culture, age, social class, religion), the type of therapy or other training techniques (including spiritual or religious) that you have undertaken both professionally and personally, and how your identity shapes your world views and experiences.

1 How would you define your spiritual beliefs?
2 Did you grow up in a spiritual or religious environment? Are you still involved with those spiritual or religious traditions or views today or have they changed and, if so, in what way?

3 What are the spiritual or religious views of your parents or significant people in your life?
4 How do other people's spiritual beliefs impact on you?
5 Do you believe in the concept of a soul?
6 What do you believe happens spiritually when people die?
7 Do you believe in reincarnation?
8 What is your understanding of why we are here?
9 Do you believe there is a higher source of unconditional love or energy that we all have the potential to align with if we choose?
10 Do you believe in spiritual guides, guardians, angels, archangels etc.?
11 How have your spiritual beliefs impacted on your daily life and journey so far?
12 Do you believe that we meet people during a lifetime in order to learn, teach or heal one another?
13 Do you believe that everything happens for a reason or that there are just coincidences or luck?
14 Do you feel that you want to be able to achieve things but feel a block in the way of doing this?
15 Do you live life through your heart, soul or through your ego?
16 Do you find yourself getting into repeated patterns of behaviour with situations or other people?
17 Are you able to identify something positive within a challenge you experience?
18 Are you busy 'doing' rather than 'being?'
19 Do you meditate or nurture yourself?
20 Do you find it easy to be compassionate and non-judgemental to yourself and others?

As you ask yourself these questions, try to determine whether they may be influenced by your generational learning, experiences you have had or people you have encountered in your own life. The more understanding you have about yourself and the more experience you have on your own spiritual journey, the more open and receptive you will be to others. As your confidence and spiritual understanding in exploring these questions within yourself increases, so will your intuition in how best to tailor the topic to your client. One possible way of developing this confidence is to try asking your friends what their spiritual views and ideas are. This may help you to work out whether certain beliefs trigger anxiety or discomfort in you, or whether your interest and passion is stimulated.

Some therapists will feel uncomfortable working within a spiritual framework, but they need to be aware of whether they are hindering their client's growth because of their own belief system or fear and this is an important area to explore in supervision or with an experienced colleague. If a client is ready and willing for their psychotherapeutic work to embody a spiritual perspective then, surely, we are doing them a disservice by not facilitating this? Referring on to a therapist who is able to facilitate and work within a spiritual dimension is just as important, as this recognises our own limitations without imposing them on our clients. I am very clear within my clinical practice on where my strengths and weaknesses lie. It would be unethical of me to work with clients when I have little experience or knowledge in the area in which they are struggling, but I am more than willing to refer them to someone else with the expertise required.

Working energetically as a therapist

Why would we consider an energetic aspect to our work as a therapist? The law of conservation of energy states that energy cannot be created or destroyed. Everything in life vibrates at different frequencies and is an expression or form of energy. We are electromagnetic beings, always sending and receiving electromagnetic energy. This energy, light or frequency, is dependent on our state of being, carrying information such as our intentions and thoughts. Emotions are literally 'energy in motion' and can be measured biometrically, illustrating how different emotions vibrate at different frequencies (Dispenza, 2017). Emotions which represent more survival states, such as shame, pain, suffering and victimisation, move at a very slow frequency. In comparison, elevated emotions such as bliss, joy, unconditional love and freedom, vibrate at much faster frequencies.

Joe Dispenza has spent many years researching and writing about the intersection of neuroscience, epigenetics and quantum physics, in particular with reference to personal transformation and healing. As mentioned in Chapter 1, he has explored the notion of a unified quantum field to explain how all things are interconnected, as well as the role of consciousness in shaping reality. Research has shown that when a person is in heart coherence (discussed in Chapter 6), it is possible to measure the bioelectromagnetic field as well as the light energy emitted from them (Rosch & Markov, 2004; Dispenza, 2017). Another key figure in this area is Bruce Lipton, an American cellular biologist and world-renowned author, public speaker and leading contributor to the field of epigenetics and the mindbody connection. Epigenetics is a field of biological research where studies have shown how gene expression and associated proteins can be altered or regulated by the environment (both internal and external to the body, e.g., emotions, diet, stress, toxins, lifestyle choices, social interactions) thus, in turn, impacting the health of the body. Epigenetic changes are reversible and whilst this cannot alter DNA sequencing it can change how the body reads the DNA sequence. Therefore, learning to connect with higher, positive vibrational emotions and be in heart coherence, even for just short amounts of time throughout the day, can change the gene expression to facilitate the production of the right proteins necessary for improving one's internal health. This will increase the energetic light field emitted to attract and manifest situations and relationships that match this higher energy. Using the breath, positive visualisations, affirmations and mindfulness skills enable a person to break the negative energetic bonds and connect more with the quantum field. This allows them to access a field of consciousness and intelligence that holds infinite possibilities and opportunities. Interestingly, EMDR therapy has recently been found to have a positive epigenetic effect; changes in DNA methylation have been reported in war veterans with combat-related PTSD (Vinkers et al., 2021) and in treatment-resistant depression patients (Silva et al., 2024).

With these ideas in mind, I often ask clients to reflect on the energy or emotion that they were connecting with during communication with others. An example is working with a client who was relaying some infor-mation to various key people in his life and, whilst he was learning to have healthier boundaries, he was able to acknowledge that sometimes the tone or energy with which he communicated was rather aggressive and self-righteous (holding a lower, denser vibration). We discussed how it was still possible to portray a point of view or perspective to others, but when it comes from a place of compassion and unconditional love, it will carry an energetically higher vibration which is more likely to be received in a positive way.

If, however, a person communicates from the heart centre but continues to receive abuse in return, then this is still important information which suggests that there is an incompatibility in the vibrational or energetic frequency between the individuals concerned. As a person works on their authenticity and heart led life, relationships and situations that are no longer in alignment with the new frequency with which they are vibrating will need to be adjus-ted. Holding on to relationships or situations where an individual feels they are being drained or lowered into more negative emotions and energy may no longer be for their highest good and changes may be required. These ideas are discussed in more detail throughout this book, as well as how to use the HLP approach to facilitate heart led and authentic choices.

Alongside the process of healing our inner wounds and traumas and inte-grating the learning gained, one way to facilitate changing the vibration of the energy within and around us is to regularly connect with positive emo-tions and healthier, healing surroundings (including nature, certain music, mantras, etc.) that vibrate at higher frequencies. It requires commitment to the self to change one's lifestyle as well as learning to live more authentically through the heart rather than ego (which creates fear, victim role, etc.). It involves regular self-care and learning to have self-love, which most people find very difficult. This is where I believe there is such potential for healing to occur at a deep, energetic level. For many, it is less challenging to continue the archetypes of being a 'people pleaser' and 'rescuer,' rather than learn to heal one's own inner wounds.

Telepathic connection

Telepathy refers to vicarious transmission of information from one person's mind to another without engaging in any sensory or physical interaction. It is explored in the field of parapsychology or 'psi' although this is a controversial area and met by some with scepticism. I have personally experienced quite powerful telepathic communication with others, especially key people in my life and I sometimes wonder if it is a form of soul-level communication where I am tuning into and communicating with another person, similar to tuning into different radio channels. I can often 'know' several months ahead if a past client is going to get back in touch, or 'know' when to reach out to a friend in need. I can also sense if someone is trying to connect with me energetically, sometimes through my dreams, and I have to put up boundaries and protection if I perceive this is not for my highest good.

Synchronicities or serendipity

Synchronicities can be defined as the occurrence of meaningful coincidences that appear to have no cause. Jung described them as inner experiences that have a certain meaning for the individual and can be profound. They are not easy to explain logically and can have a level of numinous quality to them. Jung's life, clinical work and writings were greatly influenced by his own synchronicities.

This is a common theme amongst some of my clients. It seems to become more powerful and frequent the more focus is given to one's spiritual journey. An example for me is that having decided to commit to writing my books, clients who would make suitable case examples started appearing in full flow, sometimes at such a pace that it was hard to keep up with. Some believe that when you start opening up spiritually, you become more aware of the signs or messages that the universe is trying to show you. These may, of course, have been there all the time, but a veil was covering the ability to connect with the information. Universal messages may appear in forms such as randomly hearing lyrics of a song on the radio or watching something on the TV or online in which the words have a very pertinent message to what you may be going through at the time. After one healing session, I immediately heard two pieces of music on the radio: 'Something Inside So Strong' by Labi Siffre and 'Bring it Back' (I Am That) by MC YOGI. I had never heard the latter piece, but the words (which are worth checking if not familiar) are very powerful; looking for the inner light or flame within when we are struggling with our shadow and connecting with the breath to the 'I Am' presence.

I often see rainbows (usually double rainbows) when feeling alone or lost. Noticing a certain time, date, or numbers, repeatedly on the clock, e.g., the numbers 1:11 or 11:11, 2:22 or 22:22, 3.33 are thought to be significant numerologically. Clients have spoken about seeing signs on car numberplates that had a meaning to them, or being on the London Underground opposite someone reading a book with a title that particularly resonated.

Whilst I do truly believe these experiences happen, I think it is also important not to get too attached, dependent or place too much significance on them. They can provide a sense of warmth and comfort in times of need, but there is also a danger of becoming over-reliant on them and becoming distressed when they don't appear. The key in life is to enjoy them when they arise, but remember that they may just be reminding us of our own inner strength within.

Case example: Lilly and synchronicities

Lilly would often comment about how the universe worked in interesting ways and provided messages or signs. When arriving at one of her appointments, she discussed how she had recently connected with another lady whilst they watched their respective partners play in a rugby match. They initially got talking about their dogs and then realised that they had both suffered rheumatoid arthritis since childhood, which in itself is very rare. It then transpired that they lived six doors away from each other in the same village. Lilly had just experienced an unexpected miscarriage; she hadn't been trying to conceive at the time but it had still shaken her considerably. She hadn't shared this news with anyone except myself and her husband and was feeling very alone with what had happened. Her new friend turned out to be 12 weeks pregnant, which was exactly what Lilly would have been had she not miscarried. There were other similarities in their stories too.

Lilly discussed feeling a difficult sensation in her chest when hearing about her friend's pregnancy, so we decided to do some EMDR processing on her recent miscarriage. Her NC was 'I don't trust myself and body' as she was doubting at the time what was actually happening. Not trusting her body and intuition was a repeated theme for her, having had numerous medical and hospital procedures throughout her life and not being believed by anyone if she did say anything (health professionals and family). Over time this had caused a block in her throat chakra and repression of emotions. As we started processing, she quickly realised that she felt bad and unworthy of having emotions such as sadness, telling herself she was being silly. During the processing, she tried to give herself permission to have more self-compassion and connect with her inner child within, which worked to some degree and after several BLS sets, the breathless sensations eased. I was conscious that whilst Lilly was intellectualising being kinder to herself, there was resistance in her body to feeling the sadness, so I encouraged her to go deeper into the sadness. This made Lilly realise that she has always avoided difficult emotions because as a child these were invalidated and dismissed. She was always told to put on a brave face by others. Her parents, especially her father, were unavailable to her emotionally and physically throughout her life. She knew that her father never wanted children and that, if he did have any, he wanted a boy. Lilly realised through the processing that she was able to support others emotionally but wasn't actually doing the same thing for herself or her inner child. Instead, she was running away and dismissing her inner child's feelings, repeating the pattern installed by her father. She was able to acknowledge that this was not being authentic. I then invited Lilly to imagine giving her father back all of the energy and beliefs that were not hers to carry. She connected with many snippets of memories where her father had dismissed her as a child and she imagined putting all this energy into a suitcase and handing it back to him. She described feeling 'sassy' and good as she did this. This was an incomplete EMDR processing session, but through the synchronicities of this new friend triggering some uncomfortable sensations in relation to the pregnancy, Lilly was able to recognise areas of her life where she was not being authentic. She also recognised how her health anxiety served to repress unwanted, invalidated and painful emotions that parts of her inner child were still holding onto. When looking at what had been the most important part of the processing session, Lilly said 'I can learn to give myself permission to connect and validate my emotions' which we installed with slow BLS.

Preparing yourself spiritually/energetically for seeing clients

The role of the therapist and what they bring energetically into their clinical practice is fundamental when adopting a spiritual approach, taking into account their mindset and the environment in which they work. The therapeutic relationship is one of the strongest predictors and components of successful treatment (Norcross & Lambert, 2018). I often say that EMDR is just the icing on the cake and that most of the significant work is achieved through the relationship and attunement between therapist and client.

Working on oneself and practicing regular self-care throughout the day is an essential part of the spiritual journey. When I talk about self-care to others; clients, colleagues etc., a frequent response is that people think is indulgent to undertake self-care. However, I believe self-care is neither a luxury nor selfish, but is instead, essential. If you are someone who is passionate about teaching others about self-care then it is also essential you are being authentic; learning to practise what you preach. If you don't, the words and the advice that you provide to other people won't carry the same authentic vibrational energy and clients will be able to detect this at some level, especially the more spiritually attuned clients. I try to work on the basis that I will only say things that I am prepared to do or are actively doing myself. If you can take this approach, reflect on how this might change what you say to others now! I had a conversation with an EMDR colleague a few years ago who was feeling busy, burnt out, ill and struggling to make any time for herself which meant that her energies were scattered across all of the numerous commitments in her personal and work life. I reflected back about the idea of authenticity, to which she replied that she felt she was being authentic and that she had a good heart. This is common, for people to confuse being kind or a loving person with being authentic. I agreed with her that she had a lovely heart, was caring and kind, but compassionately suggested if she was being authentic, she would not have been feeling so ill or at breaking point. Her self-care was minimal, with the occasional visit to an alternative therapist when in crisis. It is not always an easy message to offer, or for others to hear, but self-sacrificing, being the rescuer or people pleaser, much as it may feel right at the time, doesn't work in the end and is usually to the detriment of one's own inner healing. Learning healthy boundaries is important, as well as the commitment to working on one's own inner journey and authenticity.

Understandably many people's lives are full of different types of responsibilities which can pull them in different directions, especially at certain phases of their lifetime. Something to be mindful of is whether being 'busy' is also enabling one to 'avoid' certain aspects of one's life, including inner work and healing. For some, being busy could also represent running away from oneself because it may feel too painful to go within; being busy is far easier than connecting with one's own demons or shadow side. It is also possible that one may be engaging with healing, but not creating enough space for the integration work which is where the real transformation occurs.

I myself noticed that the more soul level and inner work I did, the more my sensitivities increased and my frequency changed. I therefore had to invest much more time in self-care to accommodate these changes in my energy field. The ego would tell me I was too busy and couldn't find the space to do this. My heart and soul asked me to adopt a different perspective. This became possible during the first lockdown of the COVID-19 pandemic in 2020. For most of us, our lives changed overnight, and we had to adapt quickly to the change in circumstances. All of my work immediately moved to online sessions for a while and I am grateful I was in a profession that allowed me to continue working and earning. However, I noticed that working online impacted me energetically and I would feel more drained and tired. Sometimes I would get severe headaches or migraines, especially as I was trying to see the same number of clients that I had previously been working with in person. Attending training events over several days, or facilitating in EMDR training sessions became impossible after a while because of the intense physical symptoms. I therefore needed to adjust my daily routine and create more space in between clients to ground myself and clear my energies. I also had to increase my self-care to around two and a half to three hours a day, which for most people sounds impossible. The way I managed to do this was to reframe my perspective and view the self-care as an essential part of my job, just a part that I was not getting paid for! However, energetically, it allowed me to work at a vibrational level that I aspired to and thus my clients and family also benefited.

Daily routine for healthy energies

The first thing I do when I wake up is to drink some freshly made celery juice. I then find somewhere quiet (usually lying down) to say my affirmations.

I first ask that my affirmations are valid on all timelines, multi-dimensions, realms, aspects, versions and parts of myself, past, present and future at a subconscious, conscious and superconscious level throughout all eternity. I then connect with my heart, soul and inner child and ask that my heart, soul and inner child vibrate at the highest frequency of divine love, joy, bliss, authenticity, sovereignty, grace and compassion. Still connecting with my heart, soul and inner child I say:

'I am completely in alignment with the Divine, my divine spark, divinity, authenticity, sovereignty, my soul mission and my sole purpose and I use my divine powers lovingly and positively for the good of all humanity. Every cell in my body and energy field glistens, radiates and shines with divine healing, crystalline, diamond, electromagnetic, golden light.'

I pause for a few moments to allow this energy to move through my cells, body and aura before continuing with my affirmations. Examples are given below, but please reflect on what you would like to bring into your life and adapt accordingly. As a rule of thumb, I recommend that affirmations are kept open enough to allow the highest possibility to come through, rather than being too specific, for example, refraining from saying you want a specific job or to be in a relationship with a certain person, as that may not be for your highest good. Instead, saying something like: 'I am in the perfect job/relationship/house for me in this moment' will enable you to bring in the respective theme whilst surrendering, letting go and trusting that what you thought was right may not, ultimately, be the best option for you. Remember that in the quantum field, all future possibilities and experiences exist. Learning to connect with the greatest possibilities, as well as the respective energy, emotions and feelings associated with these experiences and bringing them into your present moment means you are much more likely to manifest these into your reality.

Additional affirmations I use include:

- I am beautifully and positively abundant in all areas of my life including joy, bliss, love, hope, faith, trust, divinity, authenticity, sovereignty, courage, strength, friendship, companionship, partnership, forgiveness, faith, healing, health, intuition, integrity, humility, freedom, gratitude, generosity, calm, peace, fun, success and so forth. You can add any other qualities that you would like to increase into your life. I have a list of around 30 to 40 qualities currently!
- I have all the right support that I need in all areas of my life, that is readily and affordably available to me.

- I am strong, fit, healthy and well.
- I am in perfect balance in all areas of my life, including divine masculine and divine feminine, giving and receiving, work and rest.
- All situations in my life flow with ease, grace and harmony.
- It is safe for me to be seen, heard and to live as my true divine, authentic, sovereign self.

I also connect with my heart and soul and align them to both my children and my inner child and send unconditional divine healing, love and light to them all. Lastly, I connect with my heart and soul to all areas of my work and have a specific affirmation for the qualities I aspire to with this part of my life. I frequently share the above affirmations with clients so that they can amend to their requirements and start using early on in the therapeutic process.

Preparing yourself energetically before sessions

Before a session starts, I allow enough time to ground myself and say the following prayer:

'Dear Jesus, Mother, Father God, I ask to be a channel of healing for {insert client's name} highest good. God, I ask you and the divine specialists to assist and bring forth all that can assist for {insert client's name} highest good. I ask that my higher-self assist me with this and help communicate any messages that are here for {insert client's name}. All that is pulled from {insert client's name} will go direct to you for healing and transmutation and will not attach to me in any way, shape or form. All those who come in love, light and healing are welcome. Amen, amen, amen.'

An alternative you could use is:

'Holy love and light, I ask you to come into this dear soul to heal them however they need to be healed for their highest good at this time. For the highest good in this now, it shall be done. Amen, amen, amen.'

Preparing the clinic room/session space

When working spiritually with clients, it is important to take into account as many factors as you can, one of which is the clinic room. For some clinicians this may not always be within their control or of their choosing. If you can hold the perspective that the energy in the room is also a reflection or extension of you, then even in the sparsest places you still have the ability to change the feeling and energy in that space. Before the pandemic, I had three clinic spaces, two of which were rented rooms in other venues. For both of these rented rooms, I took in a Himalayan salt lamp and some crystals. I kept these tucked away in a corner until I came to use the room, at which point I would then get them out and make them a small feature – this doesn't have to be overt and off-putting for clients, but it demonstrates the intention of working with a spiritual focus. I also purchased some guardian healing spray for each setting and would spray the room when I arrived. If you are going to use aromatherapy oils, incense, or perform a ritual cleansing by smudging the room (I now use a black sage smudge stick), take care that the scent isn't too strong or that your clients don't have allergic reactions and leave enough time for the scent to dissipate so it is not too overwhelming. Also, take care not to set off any fire alarms if you are using smudge sticks or incense!

If you are renting or sharing clinic space, be mindful that the energy from other clinicians or clients may still be present in the clinic space and this may not always be positive or resonate with your own energy. If you are completely limited to what you are able to bring with you or leave in the room, then don't forget your ability to cleanse the room energetically with a healing prayer. You could also open up a portal to the Divine or another healing realm at the beginning of your sessions, being mindful and vigilant that if you do open any portals, you close them down at the end of your clinic sessions. An example of such a prayer could be:

'Angels, teachers, guides, Divine {alter or amend according to your own beliefs or support team} I ask that you clear and cleanse the room of any negative or stuck energies and transmute these into divine healing love and light. I ask that you fill this clinic room with pure divine healing love and light that will facilitate and provide healing and support for any work that I complete with my clients today. Thank you, thank you, thank you.'

Before the client enters the room, set the intention of connecting with them at a heart and soul level and continue to hold this intention throughout the session. This will enable you to work within a spiritual resonance and offers the opportunity for the client to connect in this space energetically too. Even if it is not made overt to them, their heart and soul will know. Throughout the session both yours and your client's mirror neurones will be attuning to the energetic information between you that can be utilised if understood properly. Adjusting your breath, body language and tone of voice can all be subtle ways to work within the energetic space to create a calm, safe, containing place to interact. Being aware of what you are bringing into the session energetically will help you distinguish what is your baggage, what may be the client's difficulties, or a reflection of the resonance occurring in the present moment.

Another option for those clients with whom you are working in a spiritual or energetical way, is to use the idea of alchemy. I always have a glass of water for myself and clients during sessions which should be possible in most therapeutic settings. Dr Masaru Emoto, a Japanese researcher and writer, explored how the structure of water molecules altered depending on whether they were being blessed with positive emotions, words, music or whether there were negative emotions channelled into the water. He suggested that the positive healing channelling of energy alchemized the water molecules into beautiful crystalline structures, whereas negative channelling depleted or destroyed the water molecules. He found that when people focused positive intentions towards water, the water crystals had a higher aesthetic appeal compared to control water (Radin et al., 2006). His work has met with a mixed response in the scientific community so it is important to draw your own conclusions. However, if you link this to the fact that humans are mostly composed of water, then the more positively we think and feel, the more likely this is to potentially change the structure of water molecules in each of our cells, raise the energetic frequency and vibration and create a healthier environment internally within the body, complimenting research findings within epigenetics. Taking this idea back to the session with spiritually or energetically attuned clients, an option is to bless your respective glasses of water at the beginning of the session with intentions or positive emotions. Holding the water in one hand, place the other hand over the water and spend a few minutes blessing the water by transmitting or channelling positive emotions and intentions into the water which can be sipped throughout the session. At the very least, it starts the session with an optimistic focus and it certainly won't cause any harm!

Once the client has left the session, it is really important to cleanse yourself and the clinic space, either with a prayer, meditation, mantra, spiritual music or using other cleansing rituals discussed above such as smudging, opening the windows or sound healing.

Since the pandemic, I have been working online or in my annexe, where I have a dedicated space for my clients. I love my clinic room because it really is a reflection of myself and I have gained confidence in being in this space without worrying about judgement from others. The most important thing is that the environment feels safe, containing and calm. I have plenty of crystals, chimes, crystal healing bowls, spiritual pictures, wall hangings, Himalayan salt lamps, boxes of various oracle cards, aroma soma bottles, plenty of elephants (my power animal) etc. I also have large red rugs, one for the client and one for me if required, not realising at first that red is a very grounding colour. Often the client and I will wrap ourselves individually with the rugs, not only to keep cosy but also as a sign of safety. Clients really love this, as do I.

In my study, which is next to my clinic room, I also have plenty of crystals around my laptop, more chimes, elephants, Himalayan salt lamps and a few plants, which stand as a backdrop for me when in sessions, again setting the intention to create a safe, containing and healing space to work in. I regularly smudge both my study and clinic space or open the windows and door to allow fresh air to come and cleanse the room. It is also important to regularly cleanse crystals either by smudging them, bathe them in the full or new moon energies or hold them under running cold water etc. I had an experience where a protective crystal bracelet split open when I was wearing it and my soul/spirit guides told me strongly that I had to cleanse any crystals I was wearing on a daily basis. I therefore purchased a few selenite dishes which is a cleansing crystal to assist with this.

Summary

- Spirituality can be referred to as the ability to be open to the acceptance that there is something beyond the physical, cognitive and emotional experiences in this present situation and lifetime. It may include the belief in a higher source, which I have referred to as Divine Source (a universal source of unconditional love) as well as the presence of a soul.
- If you are interested in exploring a spiritual approach to your clinical work, it is important for you to reflect and understand your own beliefs before introducing spirituality with your clients.
- Remember to accept and support your client in discovering their own truth which may or may not resonate with your own, adopting a compassionate and non-judgemental approach to your work.
- Signs that may suggest your client is spiritually aware can include activities they participate in, for example, yoga, Tai Chi, meditation or mindfulness, retreats, attending church or spiritualist groups.
- An alternative or additional component to working spiritually can involve understanding oneself as an energetic being that vibrates at certain frequencies dependent on the emotions they are connected with or are carrying within their energetic field.
- Learning to connect with higher vibrational emotions such as joy, love, bliss, grace, can help to raise a person's energetic frequency over time as well as have a positive impact on their health. This is a field of research known as epigenetics.
- Preparing yourself to work energetically before, during, and after sessions facilitates working with clients in a multi-dimensional healing way.

Chapter 3

BioPsychoSocioSpiritual approach to treating psychological distress

'There is no fear in love.'

1 John 4:18

This chapter focuses on a BioPsychoSocioSpiritual approach to treating psychological distress. Heart Led Psychotherapy (HLP) is introduced as a new, spiritually informed therapy which has two working models. The Heart Led (HL) model can be used with any client regardless of their spiritual beliefs. The Heart and Soul Led (HASL) model can be applied to those clients open to the concept of a soul. The key spiritual concepts underlying both models are detailed, including the idea that life is seen as an individual journey on which to experience and understand life lessons such as abundance, compassion, trust or forgiveness. In HLP, challenges in life are seen as opportunities to help an individual experience such life lessons in order to grow in self-love, honour their heart and soul, and live an authentic life. Using a BioPsychoSocioSpiritual approach, details are provided of how HLP can be integrated within EMDR therapy. When is a good time to introduce clients to HLP during the therapeutic process is explored and illustrated with case studies.

The development of a BioPsychoSocioSpiritual Model

Engel (1977) initially proposed adopting a BioPsychoSocial model in medicine and psychiatry that was revolutionary at the time, moving away from the previous linear cause and effect mentality to allow the integration of psychosocial factors. Within this model, some of a client's difficulties may be biologically based, that is, as a result of a chemical imbalance (often genetic) and in such instances, medical intervention may the most appropriate treatment. Difficulties may also be psychological in nature, often identifying the impact of attachment relationships throughout the client's life, as well as significant life events or traumas experienced. In addition, understanding the social situations and environment that a client has experienced or is currently inhabiting, is imperative when determining how much these have impacted, or still are impacting on their life, experiences and choices.

DOI: 10.4324/9781003509646-4

One of the main reasons why clients enter therapy is because they are dissatisfied with various aspects of their lives or because they are suffering, in distress, and seek relief from this discomfort. It is our role as therapists and clinicians to facilitate clients in finding relief using a variety of different psychological, systemic and biological techniques and interventions depending on our experience and training. By adopting a BioPsychoSocial model, wonderful healing can come from utilising many of the psychotherapies currently available. EMDR (Shapiro, 2018) is a very effective trauma therapy that processes distressing memories into adaptive resolution and I am always impressed at how individuals can reach a place of healing by finding compassion, forgiveness, or acceptance when using this therapy. Dyadic Developmental Psychotherapy (DDP) is another powerful intervention which uses the PACE approach: playfulness (representing a lightness and sense of hope), acceptance, curiosity and empathy, to engage and work deeply with very traumatised, abused and neglected individuals (Hughes, 2007; Golding, 2008). It is also a wonderful way of engaging with any client regardless of their attachment history. Some psychotherapies are particularly focused on acceptance, for example Acceptance and Commitment Therapy (Hayes, Strosahl & Wilson, 2016) or Mindfulness. Most traditional psychotherapies however tend to focus on the present incarnation and do not overtly take into account spirituality, quantum healing, soul level work, or potential past life issues and trauma. Incorporating a spiritual intervention can complement and enhance our current skills and expertise.

Some authors recognise the importance of including spirituality within healthcare provisions (King, 2000; McKee & Chappel, 1992), but it was Sulmasy (2002) who proposed a philosophical anthropology to a BioPsychoSocial-Spiritual model when treating clients at the end of their lives, where spirituality is considered intrinsic within the individual. Since then, a BioPsychoSocioSpiritual approach has been explored more widely, including the areas of health psychology, family therapy, chronic pain and cancer. Hacker Hughes (2017) suggested that a BioPsychoSocioSpiritual approach could be used to understand psychological distress including anxiety, depression and Post Traumatic Stress Disorder (PTSD). His experience is similar to mine in that the traditional BioPsychoSocial approach does not take account everything in a person's life, because it omits the opportunity to address how a spiritual perspective can provide an understanding of psychological distress and deeper healing if desired. Read (2019) proposed adopting a BioPsychoSocialArchetypal approach when working with clients, influenced by Carl Jung's concept of the archetype. Dobo (2023) provided a clear framework for therapists to follow where Jungian psychology is integrated within EMDR therapy.

What is Heart Led Psychotherapy (HLP)?

HLP is a spiritually informed psychotherapy that provides a way of teaching clients to start living through their heart and soul rather than their ego, so that they live a more authentic life which is freer of pain and suffering. In HLP, the term 'ego' (discussed in detail in Chapter 4) is used to refer to an individual's 'self-image', or conscious, perceived thoughts and over-analysis of the world in which they live, where subject and object are considered distinct and separate. The term 'heart' refers to a person's emotional centre that is the source of unconditional love, compassion, inner wisdom and truth. The word 'psychotherapy' is derived from ancient Greek where *psyche* is the 'breath, spirit or soul' and *therapeia* is 'healing.' HLP therefore encapsulates healing of the spirit or soul through heart led techniques that are spiritually informed.

HLP has two working models. The HL (Heart Led) model *can be used with any client regardless of their spiritual beliefs.* For many clients this is sufficient and can be used either as a standalone spiritually informed psychotherapy, or can be incorporated with other psychotherapies. If clients are open to spirituality, then the HASL (Heart and Soul Led) model supports them to honour what feels authentic at a soul level as well as a heart level.

The process of incorporating HLP with clients in EMDR therapy is discussed in Part 3 of this book. Both HLP models have the same underpinnings which support the understanding of the root cause of a client's psychological distress and are illustrated in Figure 3.1.

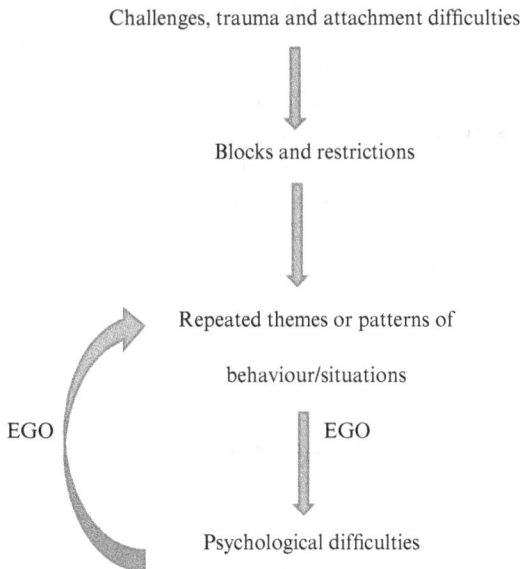

Challenges, trauma and attachment difficulties

Blocks and restrictions

Repeated themes or patterns of

behaviour/situations

EGO

EGO

Psychological difficulties

Figure 3.1 Underpinnings of HLP
Source: © Alexandra Dent (2020). *Using Spirituality in Psychotherapy*, Routledge. Reproduced by permission of Taylor & Francis Group.

To summarise:

- Challenges, trauma or attachment/relationship difficulties create blocks and restrictions.
- Blocks and restrictions cause repeated themes or patterns of behaviour/ situations.
- The repeated themes lead to psychological distress. The ego creates a repetitive cycle that maintains the repeated themes.

In the context of this book, the word trauma is used to represent any life event or repeated enduring events that have caused significant distress and have interfered with an individual's ability to cope with normal functioning. Examples include: bullying, attachment issues, abuse (sexual, physical, emotional) and neglect, accidents or illnesses and many other situations where a person has felt that they did not have a sense of safety or of being in control, or where they felt responsible or self-defective in situations. Traumatic symptoms can manifest hours, weeks, months, years or decades after the event.

Key spiritual concepts of HLP

The key concepts behind HLP are based on some spiritually informed beliefs (rather than proven facts). This includes the idea that life is seen as an individual journey in which there are opportunities to understand and experience life lessons. Newton (2011) suggested that a soul belongs to a primary soul group, or soul cluster, and that this group works supportively as a collective to facilitate each soul in experiencing its own individual life lessons through various encounters and challenges during different incarnations. Life lessons represent the main theme/s that a person will be working on during a lifetime, examples of which are illustrated in more detail in Chapter 7, but includes areas such as faith, acceptance, hope, self-worth, humility etc. Newton believed that souls work together in order to LEARN, TEACH and HEAL. There are four main categories of life lessons emphasised in HLP; primary, joint, everyday, and systemic life lessons. Everyone will have a primary life lesson to experience (and sometimes a few secondary life lessons) and this represents the main theme that a person will be working on throughout their lifetime. Primary life lessons can be specific to certain areas of a person's life or may be more general, including work, finances, significant relationships, health, personal growth, spirituality, friendships, family, hobbies and interests, environment or systems. Some individuals may have a number of joint life lessons with a few key individuals in their life where they can work together on additional themes beyond their primary life lesson. One individual may be playing more of a teacher or learner role or both and are working together equally in order to heal. Everyday life lessons are another opportunity to experience additional life lessons and may be more prevalent at certain points during a person's lifetime. Finally, systemic life lessons represent challenges or events that impact us in our community as well as nationally and internationally and provide another opportunity to experience and understand themes in a broader sense within our relationships and wider environment.

Weiss & Weiss (2012) proposed that before each incarnation, souls choose with other souls (by making 'contracts' with each other) who will take the significant role, for example, who will be the mother, father, sibling, child, lover, friend, work colleague. They suggest it is similar to creating a script for a drama and different souls from the primary soul group will decide which character they will play and the basis of the different scenes. During another incarnation the roles may be completely different but the basic principle remains the same – each soul is provided with an opportunity to experience their own life lesson by learning, teaching and healing, as well as facilitating other souls. Souls from different soul groups interact and facilitate with each other during this process, perhaps by acting as a 'stand-in' or as an 'extra part' to facilitate the experience of other souls in their life lessons which is why situations can happen in home life, work life, relationships etc., at the same time.

Weiss & Weiss (2012) and other past life regression therapists (e.g., Newton, 2011; Tomlinson, 2012) have suggested we return time and time again to work within soul groups on our individual spiritual journey, facilitating each other in the process. Challenging relationships present themselves as chances to heal and forgive any difficulties that have arisen between souls in past lives. By gaining a higher perspective of our soul's journey through many lifetimes, these authors suggested that we are able to release guilt, despair and a sense of feeling trapped or being rushed, and instead embrace the journey, learn spiritual lessons and that once achieved, reincarnation is no longer needed.

Stages of HLP

Whether you are using the HL or HASL model, the structure to follow includes:

- Identifying current life challenges, traumas, and attachment/relationship difficulties.
- Identifying current life blocks and restrictions.
- Identifying current life repeated themes.
- Enabling clients to become aware of the impact of their ego.
- Helping clients to start becoming an observer to the challenges they find themselves in.
- Identifying which potential life lessons clients are experiencing through their challenging situations.
- Helping clients to move their awareness into their heart and soul and start recognising what new choices they can make and what positives they can take away from challenges. This may require clients to take leaps of faith.

Figure 3.2 illustrates the HL model.

Challenges, trauma and attachment difficulties

Blocks and restrictions

Repeated patterns of behaviour or situations

EGO   EGO

Psychological distress

EGO

Becoming the observer

Identify what life lessons can be experienced

EGO   HEART

Make same choices   Make new choices

Attain gifts

Self-love and authenticity

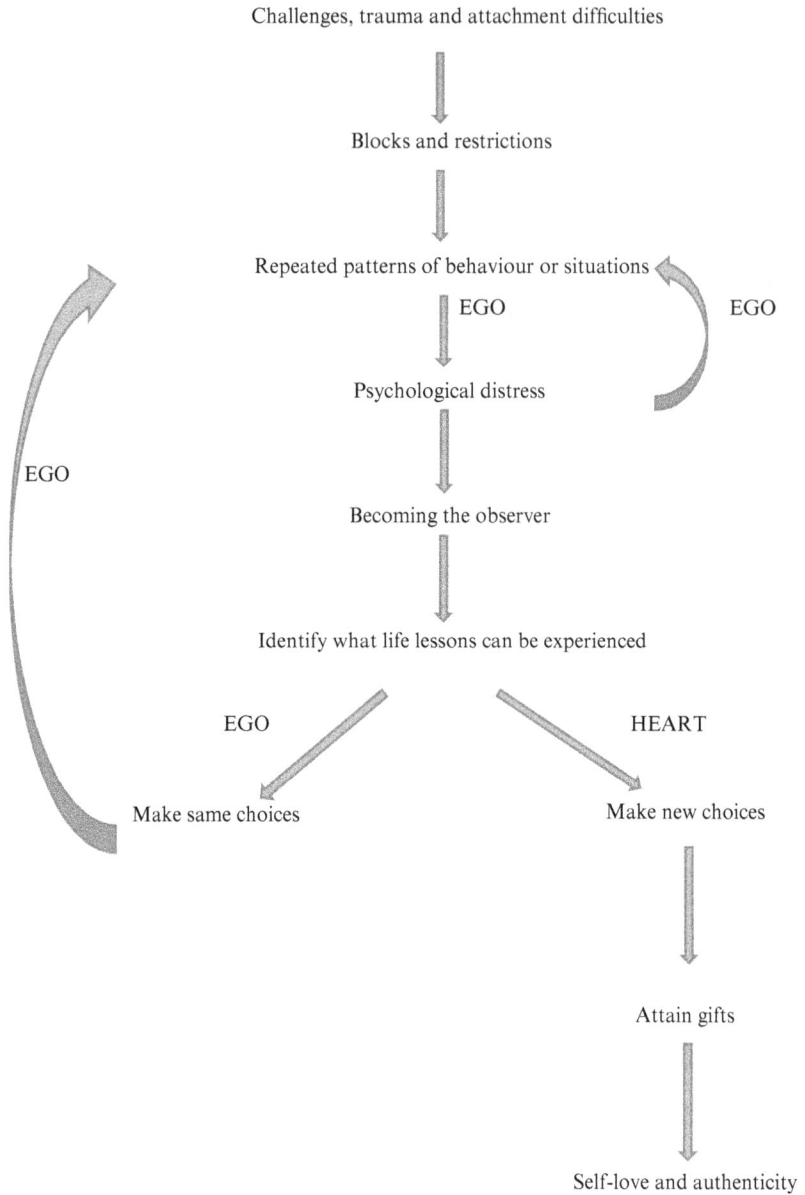

Figure 3.2 The Heart Led model
Source: © Alexandra Dent (2020). *Using Spirituality in Psychotherapy*, Routledge. Reproduced by permission of Taylor & Francis Group.

Key concepts of the HL model

- Everyone is on their own *individual* life journey.
- The life journey is an opportunity to experience *life lessons*. Life lessons are themes to experience that provide opportunities to honour the authentic self.
- Encounters with other individuals offer opportunities to l*earn, teach*, or *heal* oneself or others.
- Each individual has a *primary life lesson* and sometimes a few *secondary life lessons* to experience.
- Primary and secondary life lessons may be specific to certain areas of a person's life or more general. Areas that can be affected include: work, finances, significant relationships, health, personal growth, spirituality, friendships, family, hobbies and interests or environment.
- Individuals may have a number of *joint life lessons* with a few significant individuals in their life where they can work together on an additional theme from their primary life lesson.
- Everyday and systemic life lessons are another opportunity to experience *additional life lessons.*
- All challenging experiences, relationships or traumas are opportunities to experience life lessons.
- Within each challenge there is a choice to be made. Making new choices that do not repeat patterns is essential for life lessons to be fully experienced. Making new choices is *extremely challenging.*
- The ego is the biggest barrier to making new choices.
- Psychological distress can result when choices are made that are ego driven.
- If a choice is made that doesn't enable the life lesson to be understood, then another challenge with a similar theme will occur and these challenges will be represented as *repeated patterns* in a person's life. This continues until a thorough understanding is made of the primary life lesson.
- Choices made from the heart lead to better outcomes and gain wisdom in life lessons.
- Making heart led choices sometimes requires a *leap of faith*, venturing into new territory without knowing what the outcome will be. When a leap of faith is taken, progress is made with the individual's life lesson/s.
- Making heart led choices allows an individual to express themselves more authentically and live a life with more ease and grace.

Additional key concepts of the HASL model

The HASL model has all the above key concepts of the HL model, but at a soul level this is taken one step further as illustrated in Figure 3.3.

Challenges, trauma and attachment difficulties from past lives

Blocks and restrictions at a soul level

Repeatedpatterns of behaviour or

situations during past lives

Current life challenges, trauma and

attachment difficulties

Current life blocks and restrictions

Current life repeated patterns of behaviour

or situations

EGO

Psychological distress

EGO

Becoming the observer ⟵ Soul therapies

Identify what life lessons can be experienced

EGO   HEART AND SOUL

Make same choices   Make new choices

Attain gifts

Self-love and authenticity

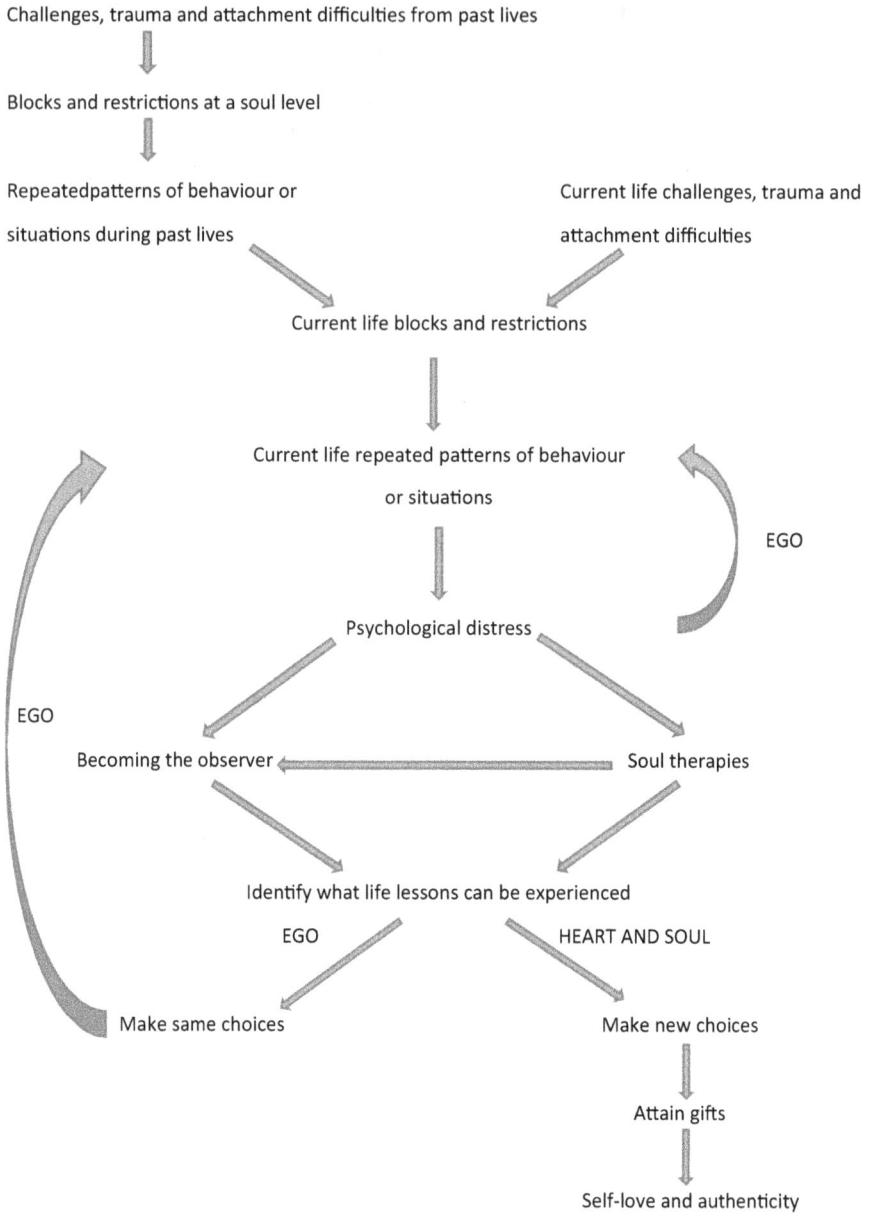

Figure 3.3 The Heart and Soul Led model
Source: © Alexandra Dent (2020). *Using Spirituality in Psychotherapy*, Routledge. Reproduced by permission of Taylor & Francis Group.

Additional concepts of the HASL model include:

- When created, each soul was perfectly aligned with the Divine Source.
- Each soul decided which life lesson/s it would like to experience as a theme. Life lessons are extremely challenging and a soul may spend many lifetimes experiencing their lessons.
- Souls work within a primary soul group interacting in a complex way, so that souls collectively facilitate each other to experience their own individual life lessons through different encounters and challenges. Joint lessons are part of this experience but the main aim is to help each individual soul experience their primary (and secondary) life lesson.
- Before each incarnation, souls choose who will take the significant role as each of the main family members (mother, father, siblings, and children). It is like creating a script for a drama and different souls from the primary soul group will decide which character they will play, and the basis of the different scenes. During another incarnation, the roles may be completely different but the basic principle remains the same – each soul is provided with an opportunity to experience their own life lesson by learning, teaching and healing as well as facilitating other souls.
- Other soul groups interact and facilitate each other and can help each other out by acting as a 'stand-in' or as an 'extra part' to facilitate other souls in their life lessons. Therefore, not every incarnation is a major learning opportunity for each soul – some will have the lead roles in the play or scene whilst others will be 'extras.'
- Souls do not experience difficult challenges in order to be punished or because they are bad in some shape or form. At a soul level, they choose what they would like to experience and the circumstances required. For example, if someone is blind in a particular incarnation, it doesn't mean that they must have done something bad in a previous lifetime. On the contrary, their soul may have chosen this so that as a human being they can experience life without sight to enable them to utilise their other senses more fully to experience their life lesson. It just gives their soul a different perspective or dimension to have that experience in a particular incarnation.
- During different lifetimes, situations may happen that create *blocks and restrictions at a soul level* – usually when a soul (incarnated as an individual in that lifetime) has been forced or has forced another soul to do something against their wishes that was not in alignment with their authenticity.
- Soul blocks and restrictions make it harder for the soul to align with the Divine Source and cause suffering and pain that can result in psychological distress.
- Soul blocks and restrictions can occur not only at an individual soul level but also between different souls, which explains why some relationships are particularly difficult.

- If soul blocks and restrictions are not healed they may be carried into the next incarnation. This makes it even harder for the soul to experience their life lessons.
- A soul continues to reincarnate until it decides it has understood the primary life lesson sufficiently (this does not always mean a completion of a life lesson). A soul may then change themes and find the value of experiencing another life lesson.
- Soul level healing can clear past life blocks and restrictions so that a soul can more freely experience life lessons and make new choices.
- Making heart and soul led choices is essential for the soul's life lessons to be experienced. Even when blocks and restrictions have been removed at a soul level, a soul may continue to make ego led choices, thus repeating past behaviours and remaining stuck. However, this is now a conscious choice.
- Making heart and soul led choices often requires *leaps of faith*. The Divine Source will provide all that is needed to make the leap successful to facilitate a more positive outcome.
- Souls can choose to move away from the Divine Source into darkness, instead drawing their energy from the environment (situations, places and people). Such souls are likely to be carrying draconian energy and may cause harm and suffering to others. At any point souls always have the choice of re-aligning with the Divine Source and being vessels for unconditional love.

Which HLP model to use

Introducing the HL model is often sufficient to assist clients in reframing toxic or challenging relationships or situations differently so that they can apply this to their life and relationships to bring about positive change. This can be done without the need to discuss the possible complexities of soul origin and growth. If, in spite of this, their relationships or situations continue to be challenging and if your client is open to the concept of a soul, it may be beneficial to discuss the HASL model. The HASL model offers an additional perspective that blocks and restrictions may be occurring at a deeper soul level which may benefit from some soul level healing. Soul level healing may be something you are able to offer or, instead, recommend a spiritual practitioner who is able to identify, clear and heal blocks and restrictions at a soul level; this is discussed in more detail in Chapter 8. At the end of the day, you have to work with your client's beliefs, what resonates with them and work according to your own clinical competence.

HLP as part of a BioPsychoSocioSpiritual model

HLP can provide a spiritually informed therapy in a BioPsychoSocioSpiritual model when treating psychological distress and is illustrated in Figure 3.4.

Psychological distress

Initial assessment

BioPsychoSocial model ⟷ BioPsychoSocioSpiritual model

Heart Led Psychotherapy

(Heart Led model or Heart and Soul Led model)

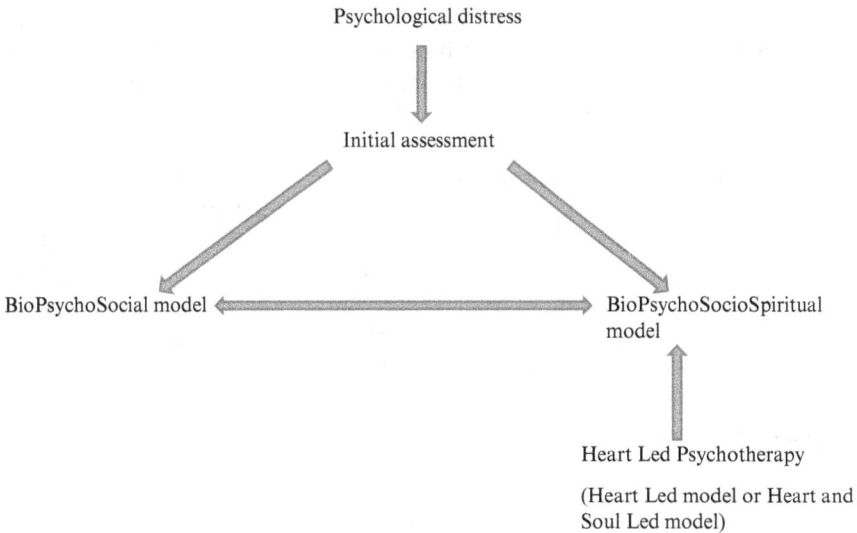

Figure 3.4 Heart Led Psychotherapy as part of a BioPsychoSocioSpiritual approach
Source: © Alexandra Dent (2020). *Using Spirituality in Psychotherapy*, Routledge. Reproduced by permission of Taylor & Francis Group.

The key to offering HLP within a BioPsychoSocioSpiritual approach is to identify clients' challenges, traumas and attachment issues, along with resulting blocks and restrictions that have caused repeated themes and psychological distress in a client's history (see Figure 3.4). The first stage is to complete an initial assessment with your client and determine whether they would benefit from either:

1   BioPsychoSocial intervention
    This would be using traditional psychotherapies only, either because the client is not interested in exploring a spiritual component to their difficulties, or because there does not appear to be a necessity to add a spiritual component (usually when the symptoms are fairly minor, the client has an uncomplicated background history, there are no obvious indications of blocks and restrictions or repeated themes or it does not align with their therapeutic goals). An example of this is with a client who presented with an uncomplicated background history, with no particular spiritual beliefs, having secure attachments yet was struggling to come to terms with a friend's death, which was impacting on his mood and ability to engage at work. It was possible to resource this client, using EMDR to process the grief which improved his mood and engagement at work and no further input was required. Similarly, you may have clients who present with single traumatic events (for example, a road traffic

accident) or younger clients who may come with minor bullying or school-based issues. I suspect however, the likelihood of seeing such straightforward cases now is minimal, as most clients who present to services have much more complicated and entrenched histories.

2   BioPsychoSocioSpiritual intervention

This intervention incorporates the additional spiritual framework in therapy and the majority of clients who seek support will have a history where the concepts of HLP can be applied. The HL model will look at current life difficulties but does not make reference to past lives or soul level healing. This can be beneficial in increasing clients' awareness of their circumstances, as well as giving them tools to make new heart led choices and reduce the repeated themes that have been keeping them stuck. If a client believes in the concept of a soul, the HASL model can be utilised. HLP can be applied as a standalone therapy within a BioPsychoSocioSpiritual approach or in conjunction with other psychotherapies including EMDR.

One of the advantages of HLP is that it provides the opportunity for multi-dimensional level healing. It does not focus purely on affect regulation, but instead adds a broader spiritual understanding to affect where clients are (often unknowingly) living through their egos rather than their heart and soul. It provides a pathway to understand how challenges help them to experience and understand life lessons in order to make new choices that are heart and soul led. In general, as I become more open to a heart led and authentic life, I am noticing that clients are actively seeking such support within therapy which means I am increasingly using a BioPsychoSocioSpiritual approach.

When to introduce HLP to your client

Detailed scripts for how to introduce HLP (both HL and HASL models) to your clients are provided in Chapter 7 but, in essence, HLP can be introduced at any stage during the therapeutic process. When I first started using HLP in my clinical work in 2018, I would wait for appropriate signs or opportunities to introduce the model and this varied considerably from client to client. Sometimes this would occur towards the end of the initial appointment after completing a thorough assessment of the person's difficulties and having established a safe and containing therapeutic relationship with the client. At other times, it felt more appropriate to commence other psychological work and observe whether it was appropriate or not to introduce HLP further along the treatment process. The more I let go of my ego and expectations and became open and trusting of the process, the more such opportunities arose where it felt relevant and applicable to incorporate a heart led approach to my work.

During the initial assessment

My initial assessments tend to primarily focus on establishing a good therapeutic relationship with clients whilst obtaining a detailed background history, discussed in more detail in Chapter 9. I am noticing that clients are becoming increasingly aware of their repeated themes and are therefore receptive to discussing HLP very early on, even when the history taking process is not quite complete. At this point I may introduce the basic concepts of HLP and how this can be applied to their circumstances whilst also making sure I complete their background history as well, so this process may extend over a few sessions.

Case example of introducing HLP during the initial assessment – adolescent

Chris was an adolescent who had experienced some difficult childhood experiences and traumas. At the initial appointment with Chris, his father was present for the first part so I could ascertain a background history. When his father left, Chris opened up about how he meditated and was interested in chakras. He was learning more spiritual ideas mostly via his sister and her friend who also used Tarot cards as well as techniques like affirmations. He told me how much he loved nature and that he believed everyone has a soul or entity. He believed in reincarnation and felt that we are here for a reason to learn life lessons. Chris showed an interest in exploring HLP and learning how this could help make sense of his previous traumas. We were able to explore HLP in our next session and I then proceeded to teach him various resources before moving on to the EMDR desensitisation phase where he was very open to me speaking Light Language at various times during the processing.

His father was aware and supportive of how I worked using a BioPsychoSocioSpiritual approach. However, I would emphasise that when working with children and adolescents it is important to recognise that they can be very influenced by others and their brain and identity are still developing. Therefore, we need to keep exploring and supporting them in discovering their truth, attempting to meet them with where they are at and their perspective which may change quite a bit over the time you are working with them.

During therapeutic work

HLP can be introduced after therapeutic work has commenced. You may already have recognised blocks and restrictions in your client that are causing repeated themes or dynamics in family relations or other circumstances, but not had the opportunity to broach this subject with your client. It is therefore important to keep flexible and open to the possibility of spiritual work throughout the therapeutic process.

Case example of using the HL model within a BioPsychoSocioSpiritual model once therapy has commenced – adult

Bill was a gentle man in his 50s with whom I worked online. He reported struggling with depression and anxiety. He had a strong sense of morals and values and when he found out someone at work was engaged in illegal activities, he felt he had no other choice than to report this. Unfortunately, it resulted in him being bullied by various other colleagues. Bill had an inexperienced and unsupportive line manager and an inadequate job description which meant that he was expected to perform responsibilities outside of his role. He described finding boundaries difficult and described himself as a people pleaser, often at the expense of his own happiness and wellbeing. On a positive, he had a lot of support from his wife, her family and their two grown up children.

As a child, Bill witnessed and also experienced domestic violence by his father who was an alcoholic. He had poor attachments to both his parents and during his teens he moved out of his family home to live with his girlfriend (who later became his wife) and her family and they embraced him as one of their own. During his working life he experienced some bullying and had a long history of depression as well as a couple of suicide attempts, the most recent being in 2019 when his daughter found him.

After completing the initial assessment and providing an attachment-based formulation, we started resource work which included mindfulness, peaceful place (which for Bill, was at the top of the mountain Ben Nevis in Scotland, which he named 'heaven'), heart coherence, heart-focused breathing and the HL model. Bill really embraced the idea of living through his heart and being authentic. We were then able to start EMDR processing on the sixth session, initially working on early memories of him being beaten by his father. We then processed his first suicide attempt at 26 years old before moving on to the memory of him being bullied at work which led to his second suicide attempt in 2019. Bill always processed very quickly and intensely using the butterfly taps and I was aware of the powerful spiritual resonance between us. At the beginning of EMDR processing sessions he would have very strong physical somatic experiences and benefited from using his breath as well as connecting with me 'eye to eye' as I guided him to tap through the sensations. Bill made excellent progress, teaching other friends and work colleagues many of the resources and HL techniques he had learnt and he became an ambassador for men's health issues, determined to destigmatise poor mental health by offering support, guidance and hope instead.

After three months, Bill reached out to me again as he had been diagnosed with a brain tumour. He was still using his resources regularly but wanted support to process his diagnosis and we used EMDR to facilitate this. During these EMDR sessions, I introduced Light Language healing. Bill only required a few sessions as he was really embracing his self-care and heart led resources which gave him strength to cope with his very challenging circumstances. Sadly, Bill died in 2023 but he was an inspiration to work with and he touched the lives of so many, including myself through his amazing heart, spirit and positivity. His essence continues to live on through many, including through this book.

Online workshops

In 2021, my soul felt guided to produce and record three online workshop videos that cover most of the preparation work I complete with clients. These workshops summarise key resources and coping strategies and are tools that I use every day in my life (www.heartledpsychotherapy.com).

The first is a psychoeducation workshop, covering the topics of trauma, basic neuroscience of the brain, role of the autonomic nervous system and hormonal system when under stress. The impact of trauma and stress on the body, the role of emotions and how these influence the hormones secreted, and how we can positively change this by intentionally connecting with different emotions to help the body heal and come into coherence, is also discussed. This workshop also covers some basic cognitive behavioural therapy (CBT) including the negative thought cycle, and provides ideas on how to break out of this using distraction techniques and affirmations. The second workshop, endorsed by Emeritus Professor Mark Williams, is on mindfulness (detailed in Chapter 5) and covers everything needed to start living a mindful life including the Thought Bubble (Dent, 2020), informal and formal mindfulness and the importance of awareness, acceptance, compassion and being non-judgemental. The third and final workshop, endorsed by Dr Steve Taylor, explains how to live a heart led and authentic life. In this last workshop, the HL model is discussed as well as the role of the ego, importance of mirrors and triggers; various heart-based exercises and meditations are introduced. The concepts within the second and third workshops are detailed in this book.

The main rationale for producing these workshops was that it felt like a cost-effective means of providing this information to clients and others. It is the equivalent of three therapy sessions and individuals can watch the workshops as often as they like to remind them of the strategies and ideas. I encourage clients to take notes, which we can discuss in subsequent sessions to make sure they have understood, and start integrating the resources effectively at an early stage of the therapeutic process. With any new clients I now recommend they watch the workshops either before we engage, or early on in the process as it also includes preparatory resources for EMDR therapy. Overall, the feedback has been very positive and clients really seem to benefit from having access to this information outside of sessions.

Over the past few years, introducing these workshops early on has considerably changed my practice from a Heart Led Psychotherapy perspective. It establishes the notion of living a more heart led and authentic life from the beginning and often becomes an integral part of the work we complete together. Whilst bringing in many spiritual concepts, there is no specific spiritual reference in the workshops and I only discuss soul level work if and when appropriate, depending on the circumstances, if the client expresses interest, or has previously explored such concepts. I am also finding that the more time passes, clients who request sessions are already familiar with various soul practices or healing and are keen to integrate these into their therapy. If someone doesn't manage or want to watch the workshops then I wait for a suitable time to introduce the HL model in the way that I previously described before the workshops were available.

Summary

- A BioPsychoSocial model can be applied where there is little indication that incorporating spirituality is required.
- A BioPsychoSocioSpiritual approach was initially applied when treating clients at the end of their life, but there is now growing interest in applying this more broadly when working with a range of psychological difficulties.
- Within a BioPsychoSocioSpiritual approach, HLP can be offered as the spiritual psychotherapeutic component and can be used effectively either as a standalone therapy or in combination with other psychotherapies, including EMDR.
- HLP is informed by certain spiritually held beliefs where life is considered an individual journey in which life lessons are themes to experience and provide opportunities to honour the authentic self.
- Life lessons are believed to provide opportunities to learn, teach or heal.
- A client may be working on a primary life lesson, possibly a few secondary life lessons and some joint lessons with other individuals with whom they have a significant relationship.
- In addition, your client may have everyday or systemic life lessons, which will provide further opportunities to learn and experience different themes.
- Challenges are seen as opportunities to experience life lessons that will enable your client to enhance their ability to understand themselves and situations more fully.
- HLP provides two working models and the framework of HLP underpins both models. The HL model works within a current life domain and supports clients to live a heart led life. It identifies how psychological issues are the result of trauma and attachment difficulties that lead to blocks and restrictions, which result in repeated themes or patterns of behaviour or situations. The HL model then guides clients through a process to break out of the repeated themes and start living a heart led life. The HL model can be used with anyone regardless of their spiritual beliefs.

- If your client is open to spirituality and the presence of a soul, then the HASL model can be utilised. The HASL model has the same underlying key concepts as the HL model but also includes ways to support clients to live a heart and soul led life which may involve soul level healing.
- HLP can be taught at different stages of the EMDR therapeutic process.

Part 2

A heart led approach to psychotherapy

Chapter 4

The power of the ego

'The garden of the world has no limit except in your mind.'

Rumi

An important part of HLP is recognising the significance that the ego has in maintaining psychological distress and this chapter focuses on the role and power of the ego. In HLP, the ego is seen as the biggest obstacle to making new heart and soul led choices and so assisting clients to become aware of their ego early on in the therapeutic process is essential. When clients live life through their ego, they can experience suffering and pain. Choosing to live a life through their heart and soul will help them make new choices during times of challenge that are more in keeping with their authentic self, helping them to develop self-love and live a life more full of ease and grace.

The ego

There are various metaphors for ego but the one I like is Eliminating God/Goodness Out:

EGO **E**liminate **G**od/Goodness **O**ut

It is natural for you as a therapist to worry that your client may take offence when you discuss their ego because of its associations with narcissism, self-righteousness or self-importance. You therefore need to highlight that you are not referring to egotism; where someone strives to keep or enhance favourable views about themselves and maintain a view of self-righteousness and self-importance at the expense of others.

Over the past few centuries there has been much discussion and debate about what actually is the ego. A psychoanalytical definition of ego is: 'The part of the mind that mediates between the conscious and the unconscious and is responsible for reality testing and sense of personal identity,' and a philosophical definition of ego is: 'A conscious thinking subject.'

DOI: 10.4324/9781003509646-6

Deepak Chopra is considered an expert in the field of mind-body healing and a world-renowned author and public speaker on alternative medicine. He maintains that the ego is our self-image instead of the authentic self:

> It is not who you really are. The ego is your self-image; it is your social mask; it is the role you are playing. Your social mask thrives on approval. It wants control, and it is sustained by power, because it lives in fear.
>
> (Chopra, 1996, p.11)

Eckhart Tolle (2005) described the ego as one's false self which has endless needs, creates a sense of vulnerability and fear, and attaches itself to problems. Taylor (2017) questioned some spiritual viewpoints that believe wakefulness is living a life without an ego, instead suggesting that awakened individuals may still have an ego but that it is different and one that recognises the self as an illusion. In HLP, ego is a term used to represent over-thinking and analyses that causes suffering and distress, as well as our self-image. Learning to notice and then release egoic thinking and live through the heart and soul may help us to live a more authentic life.

We all have egos and when I talk about the ego, I am not referring to something bad or ineffective within us. All of us will be affected by our egos at various points throughout the day, some days more than others, and if you don't believe this, then that is your ego talking! The ego can be a trickster at times, creating vivid horror movies that feel extremely powerful and real. Sometimes, I have to smile internally and say to my ego, with compassion, 'thank you, but you have had enough air time for today.' This helps me to have a healthier relationship with the part of me that is familiar with fear, victimisation, trauma and my shadow side.

Since birth and throughout childhood we are encouraged by others on how to think, learn, have expectations, desires, ambitions, be in control and so forth. It is ingrained into us by the systems around us, not necessarily con-sciously or manipulatively, but it happens nonetheless. Interestingly, as the ego strengthens through our life, our awareness and ability to be mindful reduces. Sadly, children are now growing up in a culture which is dominated by social media and technology which also impacts on the ego; they believe they have to keep up with their peer group in order to feel valued or fit in, wanting the latest technology and becoming addicted to communicating through social media rather than engaging in direct social interactions. Many children nowadays are losing their own individual identity and self-belief and most frighteningly, the ability to play, be joyful, creative, free spirited and mindful. They, and countless adults in society, are hooked into technology and more research is evolving to show the detrimental impact this is having on children's mental and psychological wellbeing. It is literally Eliminating God/Goodness Out!

I wonder whether we are only ever able to progress as far as our belief system will allow. As I move along my spiritual journey, I have increasingly become aware of the many beliefs I have held through my life from other people, whether it is from my upbringing, school, work, spiritual connections, etc. The world can feel very judgemental. I've also been fascinated by some very rigid beliefs that have been communicated on training courses, both work- and spiritual-related. I once attended a therapy training course where the leader said, 'we will always have the negative belief that we are not good enough.' I sat there rather stunned, because here was an influential person trying to teach participants about healing trauma therapy but also suggesting to the audience that they would always believe they were not good enough. That certainly didn't resonate with me. With this in mind, I think this belief said quite a bit about the trainer which they were, worryingly, projecting onto others. It is so easy to listen to influential people and adopt their belief system, integrating it as your own, especially at times of vulnerability. I have done this many times in the past but I am now much more discerning when I hear people's perspectives and ideas. I listen with curiosity but at the same time tune in to my heart and check whether it resonates with me. I encourage all my clients, colleagues and friends to do the same and find their own truth which may be different from mine or those around them. These beliefs may change as we meet new people and have new experiences and continue working on our authenticity.

Characteristics of the ego

These include:

- **Hooks** – the ego hooks into situations or people and clings on for dear life, causing suffering and pain. The ego strengthens the hook by justifying its necessity.
- **Expectations** – that clients have because they feel dissatisfied and believe they would feel better if they achieved something or had more in their lives. This could be in relation to others, objects and materialism – 'if I have a new car or the latest gadget then I know I am successful,' 'if I get the job then that shows I am important and significant,' 'if I had someone to love me then I would be OK,' 'if I do this healing then everything will be ok.' The list is endless.
- **Victim role** – the ego persuades clients that they are still victims in their situations long after the trauma or challenge. Therefore, it plays a central role in maintaining psychological distress because it creates a sense of powerlessness, helplessness and vulnerability. The ego makes it hard for clients to view their situation with clarity, take ownership of the trauma or challenge and make new choices.

- **Fear** – of being alone, unloved or unwanted. In order to heal from this, clients have to face their fear straight on and experience this in its fullest, to know that they can have love that is not dependent on anyone else, instead learning to love and accept themselves. This doesn't mean they have to spend the rest of their lives being lonely, but that when they find that place of self-love and self-worth, they no longer need others to fill that void. They have filled that space with sufficient love and gratitude for who they are, that they can live peacefully and joyously alongside others. This is a much healthier place to be, not only for themselves, but also in their relationships which will then complement them rather than place them in a state of dependency.

Clients' egos can easily be triggered by other people and when this activates negative emotions such as anger, hurt, frustration or annoyance, they are more likely to respond in a confrontational, defensive and non-compassionate manner. Learning to let go of the ego and connect with the heart is the ultimate place to be because it allows clients to be free of hooks, expectations, fear and taking the role of victim. Freedom from egoic thinking enables them to appreciate and enjoy everything around them. Instead of searching for what is missing in their lives, our clients start seeing what they have and appreciating it with gratitude.

I used to be quite nervous about introducing the topic of ego with clients. Now I realise that my fear was my own ego telling me that I mustn't do this because I would offend my clients! My own ego didn't want my heart and soul or anyone else's to take the lead role because it would feel redundant. I am learning that if I introduce the topic with sensitivity and compassion, I get a positive reception from clients as they readily begin to recognise how much of their lives is ego-driven, which has made them feel a victim to their circumstances.

In HLP, this is how I introduce the topic of ego with my clients:

'There is a general acceptance that we all have an ego. When I talk about the ego, I am not referring to being narcissistic or self-righteous. Instead, I am referring to that part of us that creates our thoughts and desires and expectations. Our ego is very clever, it hooks us into people or situations because it makes us believe that we need these things in order to function or survive, but this creates dependency and we stop believing that we can function without such things. Our ego makes us judge and feel judged or criticised, makes us take the blame for difficulties or feel responsible for everyone else's happiness except our own. The problem is that when we live life through our ego, we often end up repeating patterns of behaviour or situations and this makes us feel stuck and trapped. We are never happy with what we do have because we are always searching for something else. Our ego doesn't want to be ignored so it provides very good arguments as to why we should stay stuck in challenging or difficult circumstances. Our ego creates FEAR about change, convincing us that something bad will happen if we make new choices – this is its biggest weapon.'

When a person has many core negative cognitions (NC) they tend to self-sacrifice, remaining stuck in difficult situations because they believe they are deserving of it or they lack self-worth. However, it is their ego that is keeping them stuck, by over-analysing and reinforcing the dilemma to justify to themselves and others about why the situation stays the same. One of the reasons people stay in difficult situations is that they don't believe they or others would cope (practically, emotionally or financially etc.) if they made heart led choices. The ego is very clever; it can create scenarios so elaborate and extreme that clients become fearful of significant change.

Although working spiritually does not necessarily require attachment to any particular religion or philosophy, there are overlaps with some major religions and spiritual teachings, for example, the Four Noble Truths of Buddhism, which can be simplified as:

1   Suffering exists.
2   Suffering arises from attachment to desires.
3   Suffering ceases when attachment to desire ceases.
4   Freedom of suffering is possible by practising the Eightfold Path (which includes right view, right intention, right speech, right action, right livelihood, right effort, right mindfulness, and right concentration).

The second Noble Truth is really explaining what happens when individuals live life through their ego – suffering is the result of attachment to something or someone (desires) and expectations. In order to stop the suffering, it is necessary to let go of these attachments and expectations (third Noble Truth), in other words, learning to release the power of the ego.

How to teach clients to let go of their egoic thinking

- Help clients recognise when they are listening to their ego. This requires awareness. Without awareness they will continue to listen and live by the stories the ego creates. Teaching clients mindfulness increases their awareness of when they are in the 'thinking' mode and this is discussed in more detail in Chapter 5.
- Help clients to identify what they are hooked into that is causing their suffering. Examples include holding on to an unhappy or abusive relationship, job, or living environment. Clients can also become addicted to food, money, alcohol, drugs or excessive exercise. There are so many situations or relationships that clients can hook into, each of which will cause suffering. Once hooks have been identified, the next stage is to support the client to *let go of the hook*. Exercise 1 below demonstrates how this can be achieved.
- Encourage clients to recognise how expectations can create blocks because once a goal has been reached they will start to question 'now

what?' Living by expectations stops clients appreciating what they have in any given moment, instead of always feeling dissatisfied and wanting something else.

- Increase clients' awareness of when they have experienced challenges and have adopted the victim role. Show clients how being the victim creates negative thinking that is really coming from their ego which keeps them stuck and causes them to repeat themes in their life. Help clients to recognise how it makes them feel emotionally when they maintain the role of the victim and how this consequently impacts on their behaviour.
- Make clients aware and accept that their ego will reveal itself from time to time, acting as a catalyst to help them learn a life lesson. The quicker they recognise when the ego appears due to their defensive or triggered reaction to a situation or person, the quicker they can move out of their head and into their heart and soul to experience the lesson. Exercise 2 below explains how to facilitate this process.
- Support clients to have gratitude for life challenges by understanding that something good may come from every situation however difficult that may be. Challenges present opportunities to experience important lessons that can then become gifts.

Exercise 1: Letting go of hooks

This is an exercise I was taught whilst on a mindfulness retreat. Ask your client to imagine that a situation, or person, that they are hooked into is metaphorically resting in the palm of their hands within tightly grasped fingers. The tight grasp of their fingers represents the hook into the situation, or person. Ask your client to explore what this feels like with their grasp tightly in place and notice whether they are experiencing suffering and pain anywhere in their bodies.

Now, ask your client to imagine slowly releasing their grip, relaxing the fingers one at a time. Guide them in the release of their grip until they can just imagine that situation or person resting on the palm of their hand. Again, explore with your client what this feels like now that their grasp has loosened. Has the suffering diminished? You may decide to spend a few minutes with your client supporting them in oscillating between tightening and then loosening their grip and notice any changes this creates in how this makes them feel.

Encourage your client to start being more aware during their day of when they start noticing any suffering and, when they notice this happening, ask them to become aware of how tight their grip has become to the situation or people involved. Encourage your client to gently loosen their grip, observing whether the suffering eases.

Exercise 2: Ego versus heart conversation

In sessions, when you notice that the client is getting stuck with their ego or thoughts, a helpful exercise can be to first ask them if they can identify what their ego is saying to them. Then guide your client to move into their heart and ask for a response from their heart. Oscillate between the ego and heart for as long as required for the client to recognise the difference between the ego and heart messages. This exercise can also be done as an interweave during EMDR desensitisation and is discussed in Chapter 13.

Case example: Virág and ego versus heart conversation

I had been working with Virág for several sessions. She was an Eastern European lady who reported struggling emotionally for several years; she was single, approaching the age of 40 and desperately wanted to start a family. She had a strong spiritual faith and a regular self-care practice. She had experienced some early life traumas and attachment difficulties which she felt impacted on her ability to form relationships so, once she was resourced, we started processing these traumas using EMDR. Her core negative cognitions (NCs) included 'I am undeserving,' 'I am not good enough' and 'I deserve to be punished,' the latter of which was the most powerful as it made her feel lonely and isolated. Virág processed her current life traumas very quickly and smoothly and this often connected to intergenerational wounds which she healed through heart energy (see Chapter 14 for more information).

In one session she arrived to say that she had been in correspondence with two men. She discussed one who was a work colleague and they had become 'friends with benefits.' She said he had a lot of mental health issues and she had some concerns about his emotional capacity and ability to commit to anything more serious. She then mentioned the other person whom she had recently met when on holiday in her country of origin. She felt more in common with him; he meditated, practised yoga, was interested in spirituality and they had a strong energetic connection. However, he lived in a different country. I asked Virág to connect with the first man and notice the messages from her heart and ego. Her ego was telling her that she might be alone if she didn't make this work, but her heart was saying that he wasn't at the same energetic frequency to her and that it was not in her best interest. With the second man, her ego was saying that it wouldn't work out because of the distance. Her heart told her that regardless of whether it worked out or not, he represented someone who was more aligned with the type of energetic connection she was seeking. Overall, Virág was able to realise that regardless of what happened, the universe was showing her that these two men represented different possibilities; being with someone because of the fear of her age and being alone (ego choice) or alternatively having a more authentic relationship with someone whom she felt a strong spiritual or energetic connection (heart led choice). She acknowledged that she had been sending out mixed messages to the universe so the clearer she became in what she truly desired, the more likely this would be to manifest.

As therapists, it is important to remember that whilst it may sound easy to support our clients in noticing and then learning to release egoic thinking, it can be extremely difficult and challenging in practice. We need to support them by coming from a place of love and compassion. We have to recognise that our clients may have become best friends with their ego for a long time and it won't want to leave easily – it will put up a fight! We can highlight this to our clients and help them identify when their ego is trying to take charge. This has to be done gently and respectfully so as not to offend their ego which will put up defences if it feels threatened or senses that you are being judgemental in your manner. Our clients will make mistakes along the way, so with compassion we need to help them to find ways to take care of themselves and accept that the journey will be bumpy; guiding them to learn to ride the waves of the storm rather than feel they are drowning, surfing the waves rather than fighting against them. Additional strategies and resources to teach clients on this journey will be discussed further throughout the book.

Brick walls or loving boundaries?

It is easy for clients to put up brick walls when they have experienced pain, suffering and distress. This is a typical response that I am sure most of us can relate to. Brick walls (or dissociative barriers) become a defensive mechanism to try and prevent us from feeling hurt again. It can be easier to block out emotions and shut down our hearts when experiencing pain. It is not unusual for clients who have undergone extreme trauma or abuse to dissociate completely from their emotions and/or physical bodies. This can be an effective survival strategy and is what may have been necessary in order to get through the horrendous experiences. However, with time, those brick walls remain in place, firmly cemented, preventing the client from learning to experience positive affect or sensations. Thus, they live life in a numb state. If the client continues to live in a traumatic environment, then obviously support is initially required to help them find a safer place to live free from the abuse. Once this is achieved, effective therapeutic interventions can be implemented to assist clients in being more present and process past trauma and attachment difficulties so that they no longer need to live life in a dissociative state. From a spiritual perspective, part of the healing work can include supporting clients in understanding what has happened in their life using HLP to help bring down the brick walls safely and in their own time. Teaching clients how to use protective loving boundaries (e.g., learning to speak up for themselves from a place of compassion but without relenting to others' perceived expectations or want of them) can allow them to start living a more authentic life. This enables them to open themselves up to receive, as well as give, unconditional love from their heart without becoming victims to abusive or destructive situations or people.

Drop the label or diagnosis

This may be a controversial area to discuss; whether we should be labelling and diagnosing clients. Firstly, everyone is entitled to their opinion and it is not my aim to try and convert you to my way of thinking, but rather, to present an argument for the benefits of avoiding labels as much as possible. There are some exceptions to this and if there are valid reasons why it would benefit the client to have a diagnosis in order for them to access necessary educational, work and/or health support services, then with their permission, this can be advantageous. Unfortunately, we live in a world where labels and diagnoses are often heard more than the client's story. I personally try to avoid using labels or diagnoses unless under exceptional circumstances.

The ego loves labels and diagnoses because it gives clients an explanation or justification for why they feel the way they do, or why they behave in a certain way. Clients and their families may readily become dependent on labels and sometimes seek comfort in them. The difficulty is that they can keep the client feeling a victim and powerless. Another difficulty with using labels and diagnoses is that they tend to stick – with superglue – and they are surprisingly difficult to remove once they have been applied. Encouraging people to detach themselves from the label is very tricky.

I am sure we can all recall examples of clients who arrive having already diagnosed themselves, ranging from depression, anxieties, neurodiversity to personality disorders. Some may have formal diagnoses and may have been prescribed heavy duty medications. I am also aware that there can be a huge overlap in symptoms between various diagnoses and some may be preferred and used by a client to avoid looking at some of the more complex difficulties that they are experiencing. Whatever the situation, I try to provide clients with an explanation of why they are struggling based on what has happened to them in their lives, using the BioPsychoSocioSpiritual Model. It is frightening how even clients who have formal diagnoses may have no understanding of the basis on which their diagnosis was made. Providing a formulation not only increases their understanding of their experiences, but also steers them away from labels, giving hope that there is potential for them to grow stronger and heal.

Mirrors and triggers

Imagine everyone in your life, metaphorically and energetically speaking, is your mirror. I am your mirror and you are mine, even as I write, and you read this book. Your family, friends, colleagues, clients, neighbours, acquaintances, people in your local environment as well as what is happening to individuals globally, all represent mirrors. Some individuals in our lives will act as stronger or more significant mirrors than others, perhaps where there are joint lessons to be experienced spiritually. Using this concept and the ideas within HLP, we are all energetically supporting each other on our own individual journeys, reflecting back to each other what still needs healing *within* by representing either the learner, teacher or healer role. When you see love and kindness in others, they are reflecting back to you what qualities you have within.

From a spiritual and energetic perspective, when we are triggered by someone or their behaviour, our egos become activated. We often feel uncomfortable emotions such as anger, sadness, anxiety, loneliness, shame or disgust, and we may be able to recognise the negative beliefs that are being activated such as 'I am bad,' 'I don't deserve happiness,' 'I am unlovable,' 'I am alone,' 'I am not safe,' etc. If this becomes too difficult to manage, we respond from a defensive, victim, ego led place, typically with a similar, low vibrating emotion of anger or sadness or hurt and our behaviour or actions reflect our underlying negative cognitions.

Alternatively, if we can learn to increase our awareness to triggers (through techniques such as mindful, heart led practices and HLP, as discussed in the following chapters), and take a moment to pause and be curious to what lies behind the trigger, we start to realise that we are just being shown an inner wound that still requires some healing. As we work on healing the inner wounds and integrating the learning, the triggers will eventually subside and become invalid. During this process of inner healing, we may be presented with similar challenges from the universe or tests to see whether we are still being triggered and how we cope with the situation – do we fall back into familiar old beliefs and patterns? Or, are we learning to make different, more authentic choices and apply this to current and future situations? Depending on the depth of the wound, which may relate to many previous lifetimes, the triggers may come in cycles, giving us an opportunity to peel back further layers, like an onion, right to the core of the wound (analogous to a touchstone event in EMDR therapy). There may be further work to be done in specific areas of your life, for example, if you have a deep wound around abandonment, trust or self-worth which may represent your primary life lesson. You may be running various archetypal patterns such as being the rescuer, martyr or people pleaser, or falling back into familiar types of relationships with others who may have certain personality styles that are emotionally, energetically or physically abusive. Being aware of this process, observing and self-reflecting (rather than deflecting, avoiding or reacting) can highlight what improvements we have made and are continuing to make on the spiritual journey. With time and inner work, the triggers become less intense, of shorter duration and eventually they subside. My rule of thumb is that if I am still triggered by something or someone, I am just being shown that there is still inner healing to be done. If someone or something continues in your life even though the relationship feels toxic or no longer resonates, then there is still something important to be learnt.

The principles and techniques of HLP provide the pathway to keep coming back to ourselves, to go within so that we can develop self-love. We begin to look at triggers in a much more positive way because we recognise that they help identify what areas in our lives still need healing. We learn to have more compassion for those who have previously and still may trigger us. From a soul perspective we recognise that they are just playing their role in helping us progress on our own individual spiritual journey. When we keep bringing the learning back to ourselves and look within, we acknowledge that there is always something we can learn from every situation and experience, even if it is to have healthier boundaries, be less judgemental or more compassionate. We find that we have everything we need within ourselves rather than seeking what we are missing through our relationships with others. This develops healthier, complementary relationships in our lives and enables us to find a balance between giving and receiving.

Spirituality and ego

Below are some 'terms' that describe the typical egoic behaviours that we or our clients can fall into or encounter during the spiritual journey.

Spiritual bypassing

I suspect that this is a term familiar to most readers. It was introduced by John Welwood, a transpersonal psychotherapist, in the 1980s and refers to using spiritual ideas and practices in order to side-step, dismiss or avoid facing unresolved complex issues or traumas. Some examples of spiritual bypassing include: avoiding feelings of anger, believing in one's own spiritual superiority, pretending things are ok when they are not, projecting negative beliefs and feelings on to others, being idealistic and not being very grounded or present. People who spiritually bypass are unlikely to make much progress in their healing, as they will find themselves repeating similar patterns of behaviour or engaging in familiar types of relationships which will be mirroring back to them the internal wounds.

I attended a training event several years ago where the presenter claimed somewhat randomly that 'all spiritual people are just bypassing.' Although it wouldn't do so now, at the time this very generalised judgement triggered me because I was fully immersed in my own spiritual healing and definitely not bypassing. I was deeply embracing and working through the pain that related to many past and current soul level blocks and restrictions. I knew that several of my friends were also in similar positions, so this general statement not only felt very misleading and unprofessional but perhaps revealed more about the presenter. I would recommend that professionals, especially those in a position of authority or reputation, should clearly own their personal beliefs yet be cautious about when and how they share them because they can have such an influence on others. I tend to say 'this is my own personal belief but it is important for you to find your own truth. Sometimes my beliefs may resonate with you, but always check in your heart first to make sure.'

Spiritual intellect

I am using this term to describe those individuals who are very good at 'talking the talk' but not 'walking the walk,' so in essence, they are spiritually bypassing. They may have read widely on spiritual concepts and ideas and readily share them with others or they may be in a position of advising others in their lives and work. They are often very talkative, keen to share their knowledge and are very much 'in their heads.' However, they tend to be disconnected from their physical and emotional feelings and unable to apply or integrate the knowledge. They are often dissociative and may have lots of parts, some of which are very functional, high achieving or successful. I see a number of clients who come initially with complex trauma histories who have attended various workshops, retreats, watched YouTube videos, documentaries, read many books, use various gadgets and technology, taken plant-based medicines etc., but still have a huge disconnect from their thoughts, feelings, body and authenticity. They are stuck in their ego rather than in connection with their hearts and thus unable to discern what resonates with their truth and what they are hearing in order to fully integrate any wisdom, teachings, or healing. This is relatively easy to identify in our clients simply by asking them, when they are talking about their spiritual experiences or knowledge, to notice what they are feeling in their bodies. They will either have a blank expression, may notice that they are unable to feel anything, or go back in their heads and divert the conversation to something more comfortable. They may do this a number of times. Therefore, compassionately supporting them to recognise that it appears challenging for them to feel the emotions or physical sensations, can be a helpful part of the process. It also highlights that more preparation and resource work would be beneficial before starting EMDR processing.

Spiritual junkie

I have created this term (I'm sorry if it is triggering) to describe individuals who are very keen to go on as many different retreats or pay for numerous healing sessions with many different healers, without giving sufficient time for integration. This is another example of talking the talk without walking the walk or spiritual bypassing. Reasons for avoiding the integration include being too dissociative, too painful or trying to rush the process. I know of people who have been on intensive psychedelic retreats, attended sound healing, reiki, breathwork, psychic readings, and family constellation work, all within a space of a few months. Individuals may often remain stuck or make very little changes in their lives, repeating the same cycles and patterns because they are not allowing space to understand what is meant to be learnt and integrated from the healing in order to make new heart led choices.

One of my clients completed some very good EMDR work on various traumas relating to her emotionally abusive relationship with her husband as well as early attachment traumas with her parents. I had provided a detailed formulation after our initial history taking. I was a little surprised when she announced that she was feeling much better following the EMDR and was now going to explore some attachment therapy as the next stage of her journey. I suspect that this was because she was reading various posts on social media in relation to this topic. I explained that she had processed many of her core attachment wounds, so the next key stage to her journey involved allowing time to integrate the healing and continue practising making new heart led choices using the principles of HLP which would help break the repeated cycles and patterns that had become so familiar to her. I had an email from her seven months later; she had left her husband and wanted to refer a few friends to me. Her email said: 'It's been a really good few months for me and I've just been flowing with what's happening, and doing really well overall. You are your practice completely changed my life, and I'm so grateful.'

I was delighted that she had understood what I meant. She was learning to create space to employ heart led tools and techniques to keep moving forwards in her life. Whilst we can facilitate our clients to process traumas, the spiritual work is ongoing. It requires continual learning and awareness in everyday life in order not to fall back into familiar egoic cycles.

Spiritual narcissist

A difficult term, but one that is becoming more widely used to describe an individual who lets spiritual concepts and ideas go to their head, or has an inflated ego and a sense of superiority over others. They will believe they are more enlightened, 'awakened' or 'ascended,' may be in a position of influence in society and may manipulate and control others to their advantage using spiritual practices or ideas resulting in possible emotional, physical, spiritual or sexual abuse. I personally feel that these individuals represent a very real danger in society, especially to those who are in a place of spiritual crisis or emergence. It highlights how important it is for individuals to be more discerning; trusting their own truth and guidance from their heart in all relationships and situations in a world where spirituality is becoming increasingly popular.

Letting go of the power of my egoic thinking

Learning to release the power of my ego is an ongoing process as part of the journey to live my authenticity. It isn't about getting somewhere or 'getting it' because that creates expectations which do not work. Let me be clear, my ego still appears regularly to keep me in check and when this happens, it reminds me of how powerful and destructive it can be. When I become aware of the presence of my ego, I try to befriend it, smile and thank it for reminding me that I have disconnected from my heart. The more and more I mindfully practise becoming aware of when I have slipped into ego thinking, the quicker I can move away from such thoughts and thus, the less power they exert. I then reconnect and centre on my heart and soul, applying the various resources discussed in this book. I am so familiar with the stories that my ego creates based on past traumas and wounds and quite frankly, I am bored with them! I remind myself that I always have a choice as to whether to engage with these stories or to process and transmute the negative affect and release the narratives, taking away and integrating any learning that is still required. As I continue with this process, the impact of the ego lessens. I am also much better at noticing what I call 'rabbit holes' which I refer to as the many various traps my ego could set me to keep me hooked into a drama (mine or someone else's).

Summary

- HLP teaches clients how the ego is involved in creating repeated patterns in their life that cause psychological distress and suffering.
- The key characteristics of the ego are fear, expectations, hooks, and the victim role.
- Strategies to support clients to release the power of egoic thinking include mindfulness, releasing hooks and expectations and recognising when they are adopting the victim role.
- Clients can learn how to use loving, compassionate boundaries rather than solid brick walls to protect themselves and feel safer in relationships.
- HLP is cautious about over-labelling or diagnosing clients. Instead, it aims to provide a formulation using a BioPsychoSocioSpiritual model of the difficulties clients have experienced, offering hope towards a deep healing by moving attention away from the ego and into the heart and soul to live a more authentic life.
- Relationships and situations can metaphorically represent energetic mirrors in one's life, reflecting back what is happening within oneself.
- When a client is triggered it is often a guide to highlight an inner wound that may need some healing.
- It is important to recognise the signs when a person may be trying to bypass stages of their spiritual journey in an attempt to avoid connecting and transmuting wounds and pain.
- HLP encourages clients to have a healthier relationship with their ego and at moments when it is very active, recognising that it is just a reminder that they have disconnected from their heart.

Chapter 5

Mindfulness

'The source of now is here.'

Rumi

This chapter focuses on mindfulness. Many clients who present to services with complex histories are dissociative to varying degrees. They have had to learn to dissociate as a way of coping and surviving terrible abuse and distress in their lives. It is therefore essential that clients learn how to start engaging in the present moment and find new more effective ways of managing discomfort. Some people may hold the view that learning to be mindful is the prerequisite to finding inner happiness and peace in life, but I feel this oversimplifies the awful and traumatic experiences that clients have encountered.

I believe that teaching clients mindfulness (both informal and formal mindfulness strategies) is an essential part of EMDR, allowing further engagement for all of the EMDR phases as well as for post therapy growth. It is an integral component of HLP and a fundamental skill when embracing the spiritual journey. Marich & Dansiger (2017) emphasised the importance of mindfulness practice within EMDR therapy, providing a set of practical meditation exercises to help therapists support their clients in learning these techniques. They also suggested that the mindful therapist is a better therapist, something that strongly resonates with me. Compassion is a key component of mindfulness and helps clients process shame and self-criticism when incorporated into EMDR therapy (Kennedy, 2014). Facilitating clients to embrace a mindful life as part of the EMDR therapy is much more commonly encouraged now with chapters dedicated to mindfulness appearing more frequently in various EMDR textbooks (e.g., Brayer, 2023).

Mindfulness is literally the opposite of dissociation and is a process of increasing one's awareness in the present moment. There is such an overlap of the language used in mindfulness with EMDR; 'what do you notice?' 'just notice that,' 'just let whatever comes up to come up without judgement or criticism,' 'just allow whatever happens to happen.' The peaceful/safe place concept uses mindfulness skills. It assesses whether your client is able to connect with their senses (informal skills) to what they can

DOI: 10.4324/9781003509646-7

see, hear, feel, taste, smell etc., whilst connecting to a positive place or experience and helps identify whether your client can notice a positive feeling within and whether this can be strengthened when slow BLS (bilateral stimulation) is applied. If not, then this suggests that your client has had minimal positive, safe and containing support and attachments early in life and that they would benefit from more attachment resources and intervention before progressing on to desensitisation. In addition, if a person is unable to be present to some degree in the session with you or during other aspects of their daily life, how can they be expected to engage in the therapeutic process?

Mindfulness plays a significant role in HLP because it helps clients to become aware of when they are listening to their ego. Used correctly, mindfulness can become a very powerful resource in life. I have worked with many clients, supervisees and therapists, who have said they have learnt some type of mindfulness, but when I explore this further, I am fascinated to discover that their understanding is somewhat limited to meditation rather than embracing mindfulness in all aspects of life. It is sometimes seen as an 'add-on' to help clients with a bit of resourcing for occasional use, without really guiding them in how to live a mindful life and use it to its full capacity. This chapter begins by covering some of the research findings that support mindfulness in clinical work. A detailed script is then provided to enable you to teach your clients a thorough overview of mindfulness as well as a separate mindful breathing exercise.

Mindfulness has become a buzzword over the past few decades, often thrown into conversations and mentioned on the radio and TV programmes and there are now numerous self-help and academic books available. The origins lie in Zen Buddhism as one of the stages or pathways leading to enlightenment. *Anāpānasati*, translated as 'mindfulness of breathing,' was taught by the Buddha as a method to achieve enlightenment. The benefits of mindfulness have been well researched over recent years and there is growing evidence in support of the application of mindfulness in many different clinical settings, in different client groups, with therapists and for the general population as a whole (Ivtzan & Lomas, 2016). Jon Kabat-Zinn (1982) is acknowledged as the first person to apply mindfulness from Buddhist traditions to help patients with chronic pain. Since then, Mindfulness-Based Stress Reduction (MBSR) has been proven to be highly effective therapy for a broad range of physical health conditions, for example, chronic pain (Kabat-Zinn et al., 1986). The National Institute for Health and Care Excellence (2022) cites group mindfulness and meditation as one of the treatments of choice for mild depression and Mindfulness has also been applied to other conditions of mental ill-health (see Shapiro, de Sousa & Jazaieri, 2016 for a review). Mindfulness has been integrated into other forms of psychotherapy (Segal, Williams & Teasdale, 2002) and is a core component in Dialectical Behaviour Therapy (Linehan, 1993) and Acceptance and Commitment Therapy (Hayes, Strosahl & Wilson, 2016). In the younger population, school-based mindfulness programmes have shown benefits for pupils in areas of academia and psychological well-being and resilience (Zenner, Herrnleben-Kurz & Walach, 2014) as well as demonstrating a positive effect on cognitive performance, problem solving skills and attention (Zenner, Herrnleben-Kurz & Walach, 2014; Zoogman et al., 2014). Mindfulness can be used from the ages of six years old (Napoli, Krech & Holley, 2005) and it has been shown to increase children's ability to calm themselves, self-soothe, and be more present and less reactive (Abrams, 2008). In *The Body Keeps The Score*, Bessel van der Kolk (2014) provided a compelling review of the research that shows how mindfulness has a positive impact on activating areas of the brain that are involved with emotional regulation, as well as many other physical benefits. Mindfulness practice has also shown to be beneficial for clinicians in managing stress and promoting self-care (Irving, Dobkin & Park, 2009; Shapiro & Carlson, 2009).

Mindfulness is not a religion; it is a way of being. Simply put, mindfulness is 'awareness.' It is such an important part of HLP because if the client doesn't have awareness, they will not recognise when they are stuck in their challenges or egoic thinking and therefore be unable to follow the process of HLP.

It is helpful to provide a thorough but uncomplicated overview of mindfulness to clients, which can get them started on this amazing journey and facilitate the further development of their mindfulness practice. I used to spend a session explaining mindfulness with most clients after completing a detailed history but since I developed my online recorded workshops (previously discussed in Chapter 2) most clients now watch these and then we spend some time during a session discussing the content, making sure they understand how to implement the ideas into their everyday life. It includes how mindfulness can be used in an informal and formal way (Shapiro, de Sousa & Jazaieri, 2016). This comprehensive introduction is usually enough to get clients going on their mindful journey and they may choose to link into other support systems, courses or books to explore this further. Sometimes however, clients do need additional support to really comprehend and implement the ideas, so we may spend several sessions working through this together.

Teaching mindfulness to your clients

Figure 5.1 illustrates what happens when we go into thinking mode. I describe this process as entering the 'Thought Bubble' and explain how negative thoughts cause distress using the following description and figure.

'Here is a diagram of a Thought Bubble and this is you here (point to the head shape below the Thought Bubble). We are constantly bombarded with thoughts in life. When a thought comes along and we engage with a thought we enter the Thought Bubble (1). This thought sets off a chain of thinking that is often about things that have happened in the PAST or what may happen in the FUTURE.

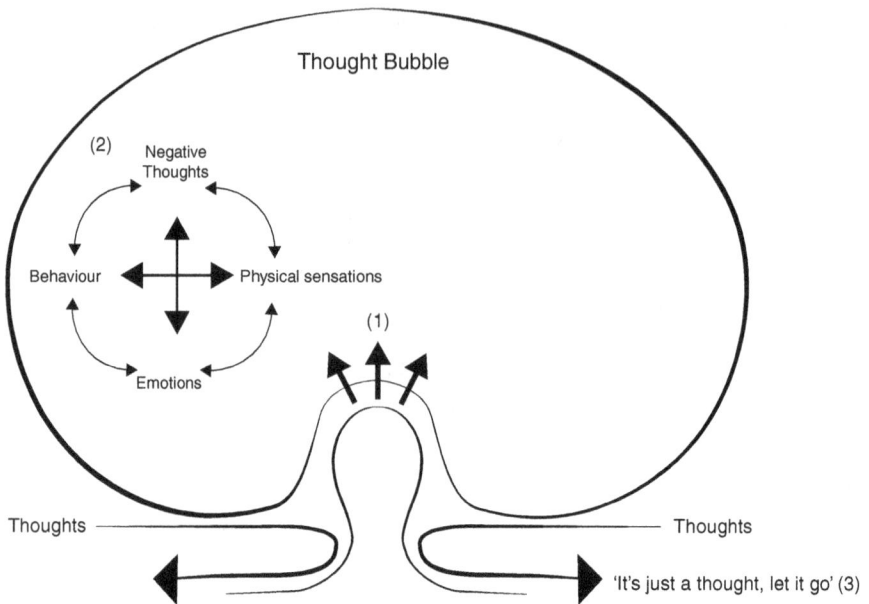

Figure 5.1 The Thought Bubble
Source: © Alexandra Dent (2020). *Using Spirituality in Psychotherapy*, Routledge. Reproduced by permission of Taylor & Francis Group.

We often end up caught in a negative thought cycle (2). Negative thoughts effect our physical sensations, for example, we may notice our heart racing, feel butterflies in our stomach, sweating, tiredness, tearfulness, low motivation and energy, or getting hotter or colder in our body temperature. This can impact on our emotions; perhaps we start feeling sad, anxious, worried or angry. Our behaviour then changes and we often want to avoid situations, seek reassurance from others, or carry out habits or certain behaviours which make us feel more in control. Unfortunately, whilst we think these behaviours are helping us, they are actually reinforcing the negative thoughts. We then end up going around and around in a vicious negative cycle (2) where the thought gets stronger and more powerful, as do all the resulting physical sensations, emotions and behaviours. Thinking about the PAST tends to lead to low mood or depression. Thinking about the FUTURE tends to create worries and anxiety.'

Take a few moments to discuss with your client how this relates to their experiences so far in their lives. This helps to make it real to them.

'When a thought comes along, we enter the Thought Bubble (1). If it is a negative thought, it may start small, but when we focus on this negative thought, the chain of thinking gets bigger and before we know it we have created a dramatic play or horror movie in our heads. In fact, we are the directors of our own horror movies. We quickly create a detailed, vivid and complex

scene of a play or story with lots of characters, either thinking about what has happened to us, or what may happen. We forget in the process that WE have created the play or movie because we are the directors. We could win Oscars for the plays we create. We are all very good at doing this, in fact we have been doing this most of our lives. Research suggests that we spend approximately half our waking time in the Thought Bubble, but anecdotally I suspect it is much, much more than this. I used to be really good at this and I am sure you are too.'

Usually at this point the client is very engaged and starts to recognise how they create their own horror movies; in fact, I have never had anyone who doesn't acknowledge their role. Discussing this in a non-judgemental way is essential for your client to be engaged and not feel embarrassed or ashamed.

'Mindfulness is completely the opposite of being in the Thought Bubble. It is learning to be in the PRESENT moment. It sounds simple, but in fact in reality it is incredibly difficult and challenging because we are so good at spending most of our time in the Thought Bubble.

Mindfulness is a journey in life. It isn't about "getting to the end of the journey" or "getting it." Having that attitude or belief simply puts a block on the process, as we are giving ourselves an expectation of what we are trying to achieve and if we don't reach this, we judge or criticise ourselves. Instead, it is about learning to embrace the journey and the ride, the good parts and the tough parts, like learning to ride the crest of a wave and move in the direction of the water rather than trying to swim against the flow.

Mindfulness can be separated into two parts: an INFORMAL practice and FORMAL practice. Let me explain to you what I mean by this. The informal practice is starting to notice what is going on around you in the present moment using your physical senses. This means noticing what you can see, hear, smell, touch and taste in the here and now. Let's just try that now. For a few moments I would like you to notice what you can hear in this present moment, just notice and then I will ask you to feedback your observations to me.'

(Pause for a few minutes whilst also completing this exercise yourself).

'Now can you tell me what sounds you noticed?'

Spend a few minutes hearing back from your client about the sounds they heard. After they have finished, share the sounds you have heard too. Often people will notice the most obvious sounds, for example, the birds singing, doors opening or closing, background voices or traffic, the clock ticking but may not hear the more subtle noises, for example, the sound of their breath, or yours, or the sound made when swallowing. The more aware you become, the more you can bring their awareness to additional sounds that they hadn't first noticed.

Once you have both shared your experiences of sounds, complete the same exercise but this time ask your client to be aware of what they can see.

'Now let's look around and notice what you can see. Just notice and then I will ask you to feed back to me in a few moments.'

(Pause for a few minutes whilst also completing this exercise yourself).

'Now can you tell me what you saw?'

Again, first listen to your client before sharing what you noticed. People tend to notice the obvious, for example, the furniture, or pictures in the room. I then bring their awareness slightly deeper by drawing their attention to the patterns or shadows of the furniture against the walls or floor, how the light falls on different areas in the room, the tiny bubbles that may have formed in a glass of water, perhaps some indentations in the chairs from where someone sat previously.

Once you have shared your experiences of sight, complete the same exercise but this time ask your client to be aware of their physical sensations.

'Now, if possible, without trying to move or adjust yourself, I would like you to notice what physical sensation you notice as you are sitting on the chair. Notice the weight of your body on the chair, is your body leaning in a particular way? Notice your feet, whether they are resting on the floor or balancing over one leg. Does this feel heavy or light, rough or smooth? Notice the contact points of your body on the chair and contact points between different body parts. Do certain parts of your body feel warm or cold? Just notice and then I will ask you to feed back to me in a few moments.'

Make this specific to the person you are with, so if they are sitting with their hands touching each other or resting on their lap or if they are wearing glasses, ask them to notice if they can feel these contact points.

(Pause for a few minutes whilst also completing this exercise yourself).

'Now can you tell me what physical sensations you noticed?'

Again, spend a few minutes first hearing back from your client before sharing what you noticed in your physical sensations. Usually, by this stage, your client has started to notice more: differences in body temperature, variations in their body in terms of heaviness or lightness, softness or roughness.

You can use the same exercise to illustrate what they notice when they eat, drink and smell, depending on how much time you have available. This can be done at a further session if the person is finding it hard to grasp the concept and needs more practice. Sometimes I take clients for a mindful walk at a follow-up session if they are struggling to understand the true essence of informal mindfulness. I explain that we are going to walk in silence for several minutes noticing sounds, smells, what we can see, hear and feel physically. When we stop, I ask them to feed back what they have noticed and then I also share what I have noticed. We continue doing this for the remainder of the walk, spending time in silence and then giving time for reflection and sharing. At the end of the walk I ask them what the experience was like. The majority of the time feedback is very positive because they are learning to notice so many things that they hadn't experienced before, and they also reflect that they feel calmer and more relaxed. This is because they have not been 'thinking' but instead they are 'being.'

'The informal practice of mindfulness doesn't take any extra time in life. How you decide to get from one place to another or do activities during the day can either be done mindfully, or you can spend time in the Thought Bubble and be "absent minded" and not notice anything going on around you. For example, when you are in the car you may notice the road and traffic, but also notice the sky and patterns and shapes of the clouds, the scenery, or the music, or discussions on the radio. If you spend most of the journey in the Thought Bubble thinking about all the things you have just done, or need to do, you are likely to feel exhausted and stressed. Being mindful gives you a break from your thoughts and you are more likely to feel refreshed and uplifted and travel more safely.

The formal part of mindfulness is what I refer to as meditation and this does require you to put aside some time in the day, between five to 45 minutes depending on what you can manage. Meditation is not a religion and you do not have to have any specific belief system to meditate. It is nothing wackier than finding time to sit in a quiet place and notice what is going on within you – both physically and emotionally. When we start to go within, we may notice some tension or stress in our bodies, or feelings such as anxiety, anger or sadness. Most of the time we don't like these sensations or feelings and we push them away and try to get rid of them. The difficulty is that when we push the discomfort away, it is like putting a piece of coal on a fire – it actually keeps the fire going and makes the discomfort worse. This is because we are putting energy into the discomfort and we become caught in a battle with it.

Mindfulness meditation takes the completely opposite approach. It encourages us to befriend what we are noticing within and welcome, embrace and greet the discomfort like an old friend, so that we can learn to sit and be comfortable with whatever arises. Emotions such as sadness, fear, and anxiety, are all normal healthy emotions, but over time we have learnt to dislike them and be afraid of experiencing them. Befriending difficult sensations and feelings means there is no power struggle, and with time, the discomfort dissolves. This often takes a lot of practice and can be very challenging to do at first, but as we learn to be able to sit with whatever comes up or is going on within us, we are no longer afraid of embracing and being with the difficulty or discomfort. We let go of the fear of experiencing.

There are several important key concepts to consider in mindfulness meditation. The first is AWARENESS. In essence, mindfulness is awareness. Practising both informal and formal mindfulness helps to increase our awareness. The more aware we become in life, the more we recognise when we are in the Thought Bubble and we can then step out of it by noticing what is going on in the present moment. Meditation is also a wonderful way of increasing our awareness and capacity to tolerate discomfort.

The second key concept is ACCEPTANCE. Mindfulness teaches us to accept whatever is happening around and within us. We learn to accept ourselves, our emotions and our feelings with loving kindness. We accept that on tricky days we may struggle to be more mindful and find ourselves spending *more time in the Thought Bubble, but on other days it is less challenging. Life is a journey with ups and downs and it is not about getting it right; it is learning to experience whatever is in any given moment. Some days if I haven't slept well I may wake up and feel very tired. I could go into the Thought Bubble and create stories about how tired I am and worry about how I am going to get through the day because of my tiredness. Alternatively, I could notice my tiredness and accept it, allow it to be within me and embrace it. Doing this will probably mean I get through the day more easily, more peacefully and I will feel less tired than if I continued to focus on the discomfort, because I am not giving the tiredness any additional fuel from my thoughts.*

The third concept is COMPASSION. It can be challenging to be compassionate to others but it is even harder to be compassionate to ourselves. This means treating and accepting all parts of ourselves with loving kindness and learning to find ways to nurture ourselves, including the parts of us that we find difficult to accept. Examples of nurturing ourselves might include finding time to meditate or do hobbies or activities that uplift us, saying something kind to ourselves, or acknowledging our achievements (big and small) during the day.

Finally, it is important to be NON-JUDGEMENTAL. Again, it is hard not to judge others but even harder not to judge ourselves. We are very good at being our own worst enemies and beating ourselves up using critical, blaming, judgemental thinking, which then makes us feel guilty and ashamed. When we do this it is as if we are stabbing ourselves repeatedly with a dagger or knife. We need to first become aware of when we do this and then learn to compassionately put down the weapon. Learning to forgive ourselves and others if they are judging us, can be an important part of this work. Starting to let go of what others think about us and not trying to live our lives by our perception of other people's judgements will help instead to embrace a life that is truer to you.

If we go back to the diagram of the Thought Bubble, you may recall that I said earlier that we are bombarded by lots of thoughts in life. Mindfulness isn't about getting rid of thoughts or never being in the Thought Bubble – that is impossible. There are times when it is good to be in the Thought Bubble, for example, when we are thinking positively or need to plan and organise aspects of our lives or reflect on happy memories. What we learn to do is differentiate between positive and negative thoughts. Negative thoughts only have POWER when we take them into the Thought Bubble (1), engage with them and create stories and horror movies. Mindfulness helps us to recognise when incoming thoughts are negative and then we have a choice to make. We can learn to let the negative thoughts move on past by just noticing them, rather than engaging with them. I like to think of a curvy arrow and say, 'it's just a thought, let it go' (3), and then imagine the thought moving away from me. I may need to do that many times to start with, but this is far healthier than engaging with the thought and starting to create a horror movie in the Thought Bubble.

Sometimes people like to visualise putting their thought on a cloud and watching it drift away, or putting it into a stream and watching it float away, or watching it move past them on a conveyor belt. It doesn't really matter. It is more important that you find something that works comfortably for you. The whole idea is to learn to accept that whilst thoughts are going to come during the day, we do not need to get angry when this happens, or chastise ourselves. We can learn to have a different and healthier relationship with our thoughts: we just notice them and learn to move the unhelpful thoughts on by. If we notice that we have entered the Thought Bubble, we do exactly the same, first noticing, then discerning whether the thought is helpful or not, and then letting the unhelpful thoughts go, without entering into a debate about the thought or needing to justify its existence. We take a step back, detach ourselves and just compassionately let the thoughts move away from us.'

Mindful breathing

The final part of the session on mindfulness is teaching clients how to use the breath as an effective and powerful way of learning to be mindful in the moment. Mindful breathing is a gentle way of introducing the formal part of meditation into client's lives and this is a script of what I would say:

'The breath is always within us whilst we are alive. Learning to connect to the movement of the breath into and out of our bodies is an amazing and powerful way of bringing ourselves back into the moment. We can use mindful breathing wherever we are and whatever situation we find ourselves in, whether at home, work or school, or when we are out somewhere. It is probably one of the most beneficial resources I regularly use throughout the day. What I would now like to do is a mindful breathing guided meditation with you that lasts approximately six minutes. All you have to do is follow the instructions. Don't worry if your mind wanders, or if you notice thoughts start popping into your head. When you notice this, just bring your attention back to the movement of your breath into and out of your body. Part way through the meditation exercise I am going to ask you to start counting your breath, in for one, out for two, in for three, out for four and we will continue to do this all the way to 20. When we reach 20 we will start with one again. You are not meant to hold your breath for these numbers, but instead just count the number of the breath.'

I then play a recording of mindfulness breathing which is available on YouTube ('Mindfulness Breathing,' by Alexandra Dent), and I do this meditation alongside my client. I believe it is helpful to give clients a link to this meditation exercise so that they can practise in between sessions until they have grasped the essence themselves. If the client would prefer to hear your voice, you could read the mindful breathing script below, recording this on your client's phone during the session.

Exercise 3: Mindful breathing script

'The first thing I would like you to do is to find somewhere quiet to sit for the next few minutes, get yourself into a really nice comfortable position sitting down, legs uncrossed, feet on the floor, rest your hands on your lap and if it feels comfortable close your eyes, or if you prefer, just settle yourself on a neutral gazing spot in front of you.'

(Pause)

'Then start to bring your awareness to the movement of the breath into and out of your body…………. notice how the air enters you nose into your lungs…………. and then back out from your lungs through your nose into the room again…………. Don't try to speed it up or slow it down, just allow it to be whatever it needs to be in this moment in time.'

(Pause)

'Allow the breath to anchor you in this moment.'

(Pause)

'Anytime those thoughts try and creep on in, just notice them and accept them and just allow them to pass on by…………. bringing your awareness back to the movement of the breath into and out of your body.'

(Pause)

'Sometimes it helps to think of the word CALM as you breathe in…………. breathing in the calmness into the whole of your body…………. and then think of the words LETTING GO as you breath out…………. breathing in the calmness and then letting go.'

(Pause)

'Just notice those thoughts as they try and come on in, don't get cross with them, just notice them and allow them to move on past, bringing your awareness back to the breath.'

(Pause)

'Breathing in the calmness and then letting go.'

(Pause)

'In a moment I would like you to start counting the breath, breathing in for the count of one…………. out for the count of two…………. in for the count of three…………. out for the count of four, all the way to 20, and when you reach 20, start with one again. We are not trying to hold your breath for these numbers, instead just counting the number of breaths.

So let's start by letting go of any of the air in your lungs, just breathing that out, and with the next breath in, breathing in for one............. then out for two.............. breathing in for three.............. out for four, and continue this in your own time all the way to 20, and when you reach 20 just start with one again.'

(Pause)

'Just noticing any of those thoughts that try and come in, just notice and allow them to move on past.'

(Longer pause)

'And then wherever you are with the movement of the breath, just start bringing your awareness to how your body is sitting on the chair, your feet resting on the floor, your hands resting on your lap. Notice the temperature of the air on your skin............. start wiggling your fingers and your toes............. and in your own time start opening up your eyes bringing your awareness back into the room.'

After you have completed the mindful breathing, it is very important to obtain feedback from your client about how they found the exercise, keeping the question as open as possible. Ask them:

'What was that like for you?'

Most clients will report feeling a sense of calmness and will often be surprised that they were not caught up in their thoughts. If so, that is great, congratulate them on managing to just keep with the movement of their breath during this time. If clients struggle to keep their eyes closed then of course they can still do this with their eyes open. They may find it helpful to watch and follow you as you role-model the breathing. Sometimes clients fall asleep during this exercise! If this is the case, gently explain to them the importance of staying mindfully awake when completing the exercise during the day, by keeping their awareness on the movement of their breath. They may find it more helpful to keep their eyes open to begin with, as this minimises the chances of them drifting into sleep.

I then use the following explanation with clients to illustrate how they can use mindful breathing during the night if they often wake up and struggle to get back to sleep:

'When we use the mindful breathing throughout the day, the intention is to stay mindfully awake. However, if you are struggling with sleep: either dropping off to sleep or finding yourself waking up in the night and being plagued by thoughts, using mindful breathing at night-time is a really effective way of bringing your awareness back to your breath and letting go of the thoughts. This is when I find it helpful to count the breath as it is focussing my attention on the breath rather than any thoughts. If you are doing this at night-time, it is ok to have the intention of falling back to sleep. Sometimes it can happen very quickly, sometimes it takes a bit longer, but regardless, when you bring your

awareness to your breath, you will be in a calmer state and you will find it easier to fall back into sleep.'

You can also amend the script to include more spiritual components if that works for your client, for example, breathing in divine love, love of God, or emotions that hold a high vibrational frequency such as joy, bliss, grace. Clients might like to use a mantra such as 'Om' or 'shanti' when breathing in and out or something from their religious teachings that carries a special, healing quality in the word/s.

For most of my clients I generally encourage them to practise the informal part of mindfulness along with the mindful breathing for a few weeks and then review. If this works well, then they may want to start building up a meditation practice very slowly using other guided meditation exercises. My clinical experience has been that if clients start to feel comfortable with the concepts of informal mindfulness and are learning how to do this throughout their day, in addition to practising mindful breathing, then they may be interested in exploring further meditation exercises in their own time. There are many different types of guided meditation exercises they can follow; I often recommend Mark Williams and Danny Penman's book (2011) which comes with a CD of guided exercises (also available on YouTube). The authors have recently published a more advanced book on mindfulness (Williams & Penman, 2023) with a link to online mindfulness exercises.

Supporting clients who are highly dissociative

I would certainly *not* encourage clients who have a complex history to start formal meditation straight away, because learning to notice distress and discomfort in their bodies is likely to be overwhelming and highly dissociative clients may also be very disconnected from their physical bodies and sensations. Instead, I would encourage the informal mindfulness practice and see how they cope with that. Occasionally, some clients really struggle even to engage in informal practice. This is an important clinical indicator and may highlight their level of dissociation. For these clients, more support, preparation and resource work is required in order to become more present. Jim Knipe's Back of the Head Scale (Knipe, 2015) is a valuable tool that can be used to teach clients in the EMDR preparation stages how to have an awareness of how present they are at any given time. This tool employs the use of an imaginary line that runs from approximately one metre in front of their head (usually the distance from where their knees are when sitting upright) to the back of their head. The front of the line indicates being completely present and aware of everything going on around them in the present moment without the distraction of thoughts. The back of the line indicates that your client is so lost in disturbing thoughts, images, feelings and sensations that they are completely absentminded. You ask the client to indicate where they are currently on the line and if they are quite far back, encourage them to start using their informal mindfulness skills to move more forward into the present moment. Sometimes completing a simple task such as throwing a cushion back and forth to your client can help them become more present in the room with you. The Back of the Head Scale is fantastic at helping clients to start increasing their awareness at any given stage in their day, as well as indicating how present they are in your sessions.

I cannot emphasise enough the importance of practising what you preach. If as a therapist you are planning to use mindfulness with your clients, you must first experience it yourself, understand how it works and be a good role model to advocate the benefits. This means going far beyond reading a few books or attending a course. It requires you to practise mindfulness in your daily life. This in itself is often a challenge, but once it becomes a fundamental part of your day it is virtually impossible to imagine living without being mindful.

Further reading

There are many books available on mindfulness and it can be difficult to know where to start or what you can recommend to clients that portrays mindfulness in an accessible and uncomplicated way. Mark Williams and colleagues have written several informative and practical guide books on how to live mindfully and I would strongly encourage anyone to read these, they are also a great resource to recommend to your clients. Another lovely book is *Mindfulness: Plain and Simple* by Oli Doyle (2014), but if you are after a more in depth and insightful read then I can highly recommend *Nothing Special: Living Zen* (Beck & Smith (1993). A beautiful meditation book for children, which includes some spiritually based resources and meditations, is *The Wonder of Stillness* by Michelle Sorrell (2019).

Summary

- Mindfulness is 'awareness.' It is learning to connect to the present moment rather than being stuck in the Thought Bubble and thinking about the past or the future. Whilst the concept of mindfulness is very simple, it can be very difficult to practise, because clients are so used to spending most of their time in the Thought Bubble.
- Mindfulness increases your client's capacity to contain their distress and difficulties. It has been well researched to show the benefits in many different client settings, groups, and ages and within the general population.
- Mindfulness can be understood in both an informal way and a formal way. Teaching clients informal mindfulness is helping them to connect to the

present moment throughout the day using their senses and learning to let go of the thoughts that bombard them. This doesn't take any extra time, it simply requires your client to notice and be present during the tasks that they are engaged with. All clients benefit from learning an informal approach to mindfulness.

- Formal mindfulness is teaching clients a process of meditation, taking some time in the day to sit or lie quietly and connect with what is happening within themselves at both a feeling and physical level. This can be more challenging for some clients, especially those that are highly dissociative. For these clients, it is important that they first learn the informal process before practising meditation.
- Key concepts of mindfulness include awareness, acceptance, compassion and being non-judgemental.
- An essential part of HLP is to facilitate clients to become more mindful in their lives. Learning mindfulness will increase their awareness of challenges and therefore help them to follow the process of HLP.
- One way to demonstrate formal mindfulness is to teach clients various meditations including mindful breathing exercises. This can prove an effective resource to utilise throughout the day, but also at night-time if clients are struggling with sleep.
- It is essential to practise what you preach. If you are going to teach mindfulness, you must have experienced the process, understand it, be a good advocate and role model.

Chapter 6

Learning to live a Heartful and Soulful life

'In a conflict between the heart and the brain, follow your heart.'
Swami Vivekananda

Having introduced the topic of the ego with your clients and shown them various techniques to recognise and then let go of their egoic thinking – including mindfulness – the next part of HLP is to teach your clients how they can connect with their heart and soul. In order to live through an open heart and soul rather than from the ego, clients have to learn to confront their deepest fears and practise acceptance. Part of this difficult challenge is learning to trust the process and take leaps of faith. This chapter provides guidance and exercises to support clients in forming a healthy relationship with their heart and soul. The idea of the 'Ful Trilogy' is also discussed which includes mindfulness, heartfulness and soulfulness and a Heartful and Soulful meditation script are provided to assist with this process.

For thousands of years, the function of the heart has been a curiosity in Eastern and Western traditions. As far back as the 4th century BCE, Aristotle was able to recognise the significance of the organ, describing it as: 'The seat of the soul and the control of voluntary movement – in fact, of all nervous functions in general – are to be sought in the heart. The brain is an organ of minor importance.'

The ancient Egyptians believed the heart was the source of human wisdom. However, it is only in the last century that scientific research has been able to prove what Aristotle knew all along. In the 1960s and 1970s, John and Beatrice Lacey became recognised as leading researchers in examining the interactions between the brain and the heart from a psychophysiological perspective. Neurocardiological research discovered that the heart has its own complex neural network, with Armour (1991, 2008) proposing that the heart has its own brain and nervous system with as many as 40,000 neurones. McCraty (2003, p. 3) said the heart behaves as a 'sophisticated information encoding and processing centre that enables it to learn, remember, and make independent functional decisions that do no not involve the cerebral cortex'. This is now referred to as the heart-brain consisting of a complex network of

DOI: 10.4324/9781003509646-8

ganglia, proteins, neurotransmitters and support cells. We now know that the heart is able to function independently from the brain. It can initiate its own rhythms because its neuronal network is completely separate from the brain's descending sympathetic and parasympathetic control (Dispenza, 2017). The heart contains nerves from both the sympathetic and parasympathetic branches of the autonomic nervous system (ANS) so will be impacted by any changes in these as well as any emotion felt.

Often, we identify the heart with its physical structure but from a spiritual perspective, it is located in the heart chakra. A chakra can be described as an energy centre in the body through which energy flows; it is believed that there are seven main chakras in the physical body that are thought to transform psychophysical energy into spiritual energy (Johari, 2000). The heart chakra is the fourth chakra in the body located at the exact centre of the chest which represents a person's emotional centre, the source of unconditional love, compassion, inner truth, authenticity and 'the centre of emotional empowerment' (O'Malley, 2018). Dispenza (2017) aligned emotions such as joy, love, bliss, compassion and gratitude with the heart centre, where one is able to move from a state of selfishness to selflessness. It is believed to represent the origin of divinity. McClintock (2015) reported the possibility of deep healing of one's spiritual heart. The heart is considered the meeting place where physical and spiritual integrate, heaven and earth come together, and where alchemy is possible.

Wilber (2000) described communications from the soul as 'whispers of the soul,' believing that messages represented opportunities to connect with the higher self and facilitate healing. This can be a very personal experience, perhaps described as an awareness of a presence within, that is connected to a higher source or a 'knowing.' Different forms of 'knowing' or intuition were described by Braud and Anderson (2002) as ranging from visual, auditory, kinaesthetic, proprioceptive and direct knowing, which can be developed through one's own personal spiritual practice, including meditation and training. My 'knowings' have strengthened over time. Sometimes I get tingly sensations in my head when I connect at a very deep level or as confirmation of something my client or I say that has significant meaning. I often know what my client will say before they do, especially during the desensitisation phase of EMDR. I sometimes get visual messages but most come through in the form of claircognizance.

Teaching clients to live life through the heart and soul ultimately means assisting them with relinquishing their ego, expectations, desires, ambitions and needs. When clients can move into their heart and soul and start listening to what their heart and soul is trying to communicate to them, they realise that they have all the answers within themselves to start living a more authentic life. I believe that learning to connect with my soul has helped me to connect with the Divine and universal support team, guiding me on my spiritual path both personally and clinically and I have also witnessed this process with numerous clients who embrace a heart and soulful life.

Benefits of connecting with the heart and soul

HLP aims to assist clients in forming a stronger connection with their heart and soul. When using HLP it is important to ask yourself as a therapist whether you know how to connect with your own heart and soul. Are you a good role model for your clients to help support them through this process? When Siegel (2013) investigated spiritual resonance within therapists, she found that some reported connecting with their clients 'heart to heart.' One therapist described this spiritual resonance as creating a heart loop, where he observed light shining from his heart to his client's heart, facilitating the release of energy blocks. Other therapists recognised themselves as a vessel or channel for spiritual resonance and some reported awareness of a soul consciousness within their clients, where they were starting to awaken to their spirituality and become more engaged in spiritual activities beyond the therapeutic work. Therapists also noticed how their client's hearts were opening up more generally in their lives to make healthier changes and choices, including embracing various spiritual practices.

The advancement in modern technology has also supported the benefits of living a heartful life. Heartmath is a biofeedback system that was founded by Doc Childre in 1991 to bridge the intuitive connection between heart and mind, enabling self-regulation of emotions and behaviours. Heartmath's aim is to help individuals to connect with their hearts to improve human interactions and create a more compassionate world. The research involves measuring heart rate coherence using the Inner Balance Coherence biofeedback system. Heart rate coherence is the pattern of heart rate variability (HRV, the variance in time between heart beats) and measures the changes in heart rate as it becomes in synch with the breath. In other words, it is the harmonious and synchronised pattern of activity in the heart's electromagnetic field. Dispenza (2017) reported that as individuals learn to open up and deepen the relationship with their hearts, regulate their breath and connect to high frequency emotions such as joy, bliss, grace, love, compassion and gratitude, their heart begins to beat with higher levels of coherence. Childre & McCraty (2002) and Dispenza (2017) demonstrated that some individuals reported feelings of transcendence and deep connection with the creator during optimal cardiac activity. Research using Heartmath continues to illustrate that as individuals practise heart coherence, their stress levels decrease, resilience strengthens and they are able to link into their natural intuition to make more healthy choices in their lives, including connecting to the unified quantum field to access higher guidance and wisdom as well as their heart's intelligence and intuition.

McCraty et al. (1998) discovered that the heart can produce the highest emissions of electromagnetic energy from the body which can be felt by others, regardless of whether touch is involved. Dispenza (2017) believed that the electromagnetic fields emitted from the human body and heart are able to interact with external fields in the environment, including the Earth's geomagnetic field and other energy fields and when they resonate with each other this can facilitate healing, transformation and enhanced states of consciousness. He also found that the magnetic field within and beyond an individual who is in heart coherence and balance has an impact on the heart of other individuals, even if they are in different locations. Dispenza's findings along with data from the HeartMath Global Coherence Initiative suggests that there may be an invisible field that enables information to be transmitted to all living things including collective human consciousness. This energy field has the ability to influence people's behaviours, thoughts, emotions, conscious and unconscious thoughts which of course can be both positive or negative depending on the emotional or cognitive frequency to which a person is connecting. It may explain why, even during online sessions, a strong therapeutic relationship and spiritual resonance between therapist and client can be highly transformative. The idea of an electromagnetic invisible field also led to global meditations being organised, initiated by Project Coherence in 2015 where over 6,000 individuals connected online during heart meditations with the intention of manifesting a more peaceful world. Since then, the popularity of group heart meditations with similar goals have increased globally, especially, but not exclusively, during times of conflict or trauma.

Teaching your clients strategies to connect with their heart and soul

The next part of this chapter provides a range of practical exercises and meditations that you can use with your client to help them connect with their heart and soul. For many clients, this will feel rather new, because they are so used to living in their own 'Thought Bubble' and listening to their ego, but as they practise these strategies, they will start to recognise the benefits and actually want to make changes in their life which are more in keeping with their authenticity.

Exercise 4: Bringing awareness into the heart and soul

When a client is struggling to make an important decision that is causing them discomfort or suffering, I use this exercise to teach them to start moving away from their ego and connect with their heart and soul. It is different to Exercise 2 (Chapter 4) where a conversation can be had between the ego and heart, because it encourages clients to stay within their heart and soul and consider different options to a situation as they rest there. When clients learn to bring their awareness to these areas they can connect with different scenarios and observe how their body or heart changes, either physically or emotionally, which can guide them in decision-making. For simplicity's sake, I refer to the heart with clients as the place in their body that is their source of unconditional love, compassion, authenticity, and, their emotional centre. If in doubt, or if this does not resonate with your client, ask them what their heart represents to them, making sure this is not coming from their ego. When a client is open to the concept of a soul, this may represent the place where they feel connected to their higher self, essence, their intuition or just a 'knowing.' For each person it may represent something slightly different so try to be open to what is true to your client rather than imposing your own views.

The instructions for this exercise are as follows:

'What I would like you to do is bring your awareness into your heart area. The heart area may represent your source of unconditional love, compassion and your truth. Just rest there for a moment and start to feel connected to this place.'

(Pause)

'When you are ready, I would like you to bring to mind the first scenario that you were considering.'

(Pause)

'Notice any changes in your body or feelings as you are considering this scenario from your heart.'

(Pause)

'Now what I would like you to do is bring to mind the other scenario that you were considering.'

(Pause)

'Now move your awareness into your heart area and just settle there again for a moment.'

(Pause)

'Notice any changes in your body or feelings as you are considering this alternative option.'

(Pause)

'What did you notice happen when you considered either option?'

Allow your client time to feed back to you what they noticed in their body and emotions as they considered both scenarios from their heart and ask them to reflect on what the exercise was like for them.

Adding the soul

If your client is open to the concept of a soul, I would add this into the exercise as follows:

'What I would like you to do is bring your awareness into your heart and soul area. The heart area may represent your source of unconditional love, compassion and your truth. Your soul area may be that place in you that is your intuitive self, your connection with your higher self, essence or just a knowing. Just rest there for a moment and start to feel really connected to this space.'

(Pause)

'When you are ready, I would like you to bring up the first scenario that you were considering.'

(Pause)

'Notice any changes in your body or feelings as you are considering this option.'

(Pause)

'Now what I would like you to do is bring to awareness the other scenario that you were considering.'

(Pause)

'Now move your awareness into your heart and soul areas and just settle there again for a moment.'

(Pause)

'Notice any changes in your body or feelings as you are considering this alternative option.'

(Pause)

'What did you notice happen when you considered either option?'

Allow your client time to feed back what they noticed in their body and emotions as they considered both scenarios and ask them to reflect on what that exercise was like for them. You can of course just do this for the soul area if your client wishes – remember to ask them what they would prefer.

The Ful Trilogy

As my passion for mindfulness and my ability to meditate has developed over the years, I could not help but notice the whispers of my soul. Some mindfulness teachings do not openly recognise the concept of a soul, perhaps referring to this presence as a consciousness in the here and now.

Whilst I discussed this with some mindfulness teachers, I was not actively encouraged to explore this, instead being guided to focus on the here and now. However, my awareness of my soul was so powerful that I could not ignore its existence. I believe my soul communicates to me at a profound level from both a physical feeling and an emotional sense. By starting to listen to my soul I have learnt to make many changes in my life and I feel my connection with my soul has strengthened through this process. Listening to my soul has been a huge part of my spiritual journey and has ultimately led me to introduce spirituality into my clinical work as well as all other aspects of my life. If I hadn't listened to my soul, neither of my books would ever have been written!

Learning to live an authentic life often requires us to be mindful, heartful and/or soulful as illustrated in Figure 6.1. I don't want anyone to suggest that what I am saying is that if you don't recognise or acknowledge the presence of a soul then you cannot be authentic because this is not true, authenticity comes from living a heart led life. For some, acknowledging the presence of their soul will be very powerful and just adds another dimension to work with in the process of healing and becoming more authentic.

The process of being heartful and soulful is very similar to being mindful. One could argue that mindfulness incorporates heartfulness and isn't a separate experience. The reason why I have called it the Ful Trilogy is that HLP requires that your clients move specifically into their heart to connect with their heart's wisdom and guidance rather than anywhere else in their body and then to start noticing what feels right when they rest in this place. Soulfulness does the same – some clients may not comprehend or connect with the presence of a soul and that is absolutely fine; honour what is right to them.

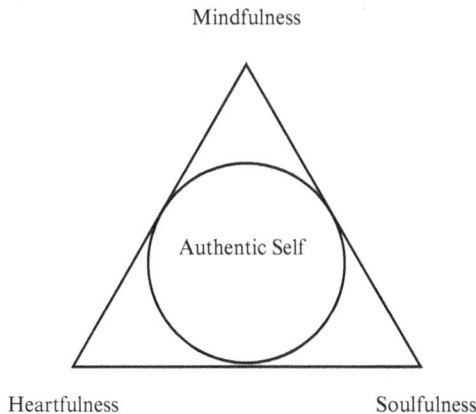

Figure 6.1 The Ful Trilogy

Source: © Alexandra Dent (2020). *Using Spirituality in Psychotherapy*, Routledge. Reproduced by permission of Taylor & Francis Group.

In addition to mindful breathing, your clients may find it helpful to use a Heartful and Soulful meditation (both available on my YouTube channel; Hea rtful Meditation by Alexandra Dent; Soulful Meditation by Alexandra Dent) so that they can start to experience what it is like when connecting with their hearts and souls. The more aware they become, the easier they will find it to move away from their ego and start utilising the strategies of HLP. A Heartful and Soulful Meditation script is provided below to use with your clients so that you can make your own recording if your clients prefer to hear your voice.

Heartful Meditation

The Heartful Meditation exercise is similar to the Loving Kindness Meditation (The Happy Buddha, 2015) or the Befriending Meditation (Williams & Penman, 2011). In each of these there are five optional stages where a few phrases are held in mind whilst being connected to the heart area (as described in Exercise 4). The phrases in Heartful Meditation are:

> May I be open to giving and receiving love,
> may I be free from suffering and pain,
> may I live a life of grace and compassion.

In the first stage, the client is asked to connect to their heart area and bring to mind the above phrases whilst thinking of themselves. The second is to repeat the phrases whilst thinking of a close person who has shown them unconditional love. The third stage is to repeat the phrases whilst thinking of a neutral person (someone they may see at the supermarket or when out walking, but with whom they do not have any personal connection) and the fourth stage is to repeat the phrases whilst thinking of someone who has caused them discomfort or suffering. Finally, the phrases are repeated and may be extended as far as the mind will allow to include all living beings, creatures and life on the planet and in the universe. At the beginning, some clients will only be able to manage to complete the first stage and this is absolutely fine. They mustn't feel any pressure to push themselves further than they feel able at any given point or it defeats the purpose of the exercise. With time, they may be able to extend these wishes to other people. By doing this, it allows their heart to open up so that they can learn to give as well as receive unconditional love.

Exercise 5: Heartful Meditation script

'The first thing I would like you to do is to find somewhere quiet to sit for the next few minutes, get yourself into a really nice comfortable position sitting down, legs uncrossed, feet on the floor, rest your hands on your lap and if it feels comfortable close your eyes or, if you prefer, just settle yourself on a neutral gazing spot in front of you.'

(Pause)

'Then start to bring your awareness to the movement of the breath into and out of your body............ notice how the air enters your nose into your lungs............ and then back out from your lungs through your nose into the room again............ Don't try to speed it up or slow it down, just allow it to be whatever it needs to be in this moment in time.'

(Pause)

'Allow the breath to anchor you in this moment.'

(Pause)

'Any time those thoughts try and creep on in, just notice them and accept them and just allow them to pass on by............ bringing your awareness back to the movement of the breath into and out of your body.'

(Pause)

'When you are ready, bring your awareness into your heart area and just rest there for a few moments. The heart area may represent your source of unconditional love, compassion and your truth. Notice whether there is any discomfort or tension or perhaps a sense of calmness and peace. Just allow whatever to come up to come up without judgement or criticism, using your breath to breathe into your heart area.'

(Pause)

'Connecting with your heart area, bring up the phrases:

May I be open to giving and receiving love,
may I be free from suffering and pain,
may I live a life of grace and compassion.

Imagine each of these phrases gently dropping into your heart area. Be aware of whether there is any resistance or tension as you do this and using your breath, see whether you can embrace these sensations with loving kindness and acceptance.'

(Pause)

'Remaining connected to your heart area, if you so choose, bring to mind a close friend or family member who has shown you unconditional love in your life. Notice any sensations that arise and just accept these as true to you in this moment, without censure or judgement.'

(Pause)

'When you are ready and feel connected to this person, offer them the following phrases:

May you be open to giving and receiving love,
may you be free from suffering and pain,
may you live a life of grace and compassion.

Imagine each of these phrases gently dropping into your heart area. Be aware of whether there is any resistance or tension as you do this and using your breath, see whether you can embrace these sensations with loving kindness and acceptance.'

(Pause)

'Still connected to your heart area, and if you so choose, bring to mind someone who is neutral in your life. This may be someone you notice when travelling to work, in the supermarket, or when you are out walking. Just like you, they too may wish for a calm life, free from suffering and pain. Notice any sensations that arise as you bring this person to mind and just accept these as true to you in this moment, without censure or judgement.'

(Pause)

'When you are ready and feel connected to this person, offer them the following phrases:

May you be open to giving and receiving love,
may you be free from suffering and pain,
may you live a life of grace and compassion.

Imagine each of these phrases gently dropping into your heart area. Again, just be aware of whether there is any resistance or tension as you do this and using your breath, see whether you can embrace these sensations with loving kindness and acceptance.'

(Pause)

'Remaining connected to your heart area, the next part is to bring to mind someone who has upset you or caused suffering or discomfort to you. Just like you, they too may wish for a calm life, free from suffering and pain. Notice any sensations that arise as you bring this person to mind and just accept these as true to you in this moment, without censure or judgement. If this is too difficult, then just bring your awareness back to your breath.'

(Pause)

'If you feel able to continue, when you are ready and feel connected to this person, offer them the following phrases:

May you be open to giving and receiving love,
may you be free from suffering and pain,
may you live a life of grace and compassion.

Imagine each of these phrases gently dropping into your heart area. Just be aware of whether there is any resistance or tension as you do this and using your breath, see whether you can embrace these sensations with loving kindness and acceptance.'

(Pause)

'Finally, connecting to your heart area, and if you so choose, we are going to extend this heartful meditation as far as you feel able, to everyone in your street, home town, county, country, the entire planet and universe. This can include all living creatures. Just like you, they too may wish for a calm life, free from suffering and pain. Notice any sensations that arise as you extend your mind as far as you feel able and just accept these as true to you in this moment, without censure or judgement.'

(Pause)

'When you are ready and feel connected to every living being and creature that you wish to include, offer them the following phrases:

May you be open to giving and receiving love,
may you be free from suffering and pain,
may you live a life of grace and compassion.

Imagine each of these phrases gently dropping into your heart area. Again, just be aware of whether there is any resistance or tension as you do this and using your breath see whether you can embrace these sensations with loving kindness and acceptance.'

(Pause)

'Now for a few minutes, bring your awareness back to your breath and the movement of the breath into and out of your body.'

(Pause)

'And then wherever you are with the movement of the breath, just start bringing your awareness to how your body is sitting on the chair, your feet resting on the floor, your hands resting on your lap. Notice the temperature of the air on your skin............ start wiggling your fingers and your toes............ and in your own time start opening up your eyes, bringing your awareness back into the room.'

Soulful Meditation

The Soulful Meditation is similar to the Heartful Meditation but this time connecting at a soul level. This may be a particular place in the body, all over, or just an awareness of the presence of the higher sense, essence, a sense of 'knowing' or 'intuition' at a soul level. It is important not to force anything to happen, just connect with whatever comes up at a soul level. This can be further extended to connecting to a higher source, whether it is the Divine Source, God, one's own personal team of guides, teachers, helpers and angels. It is important to make sure the intention is set to only ask for support and guidance that comes from a loving, positive source which is for the highest good.

As with the Heartful Meditation, there are five optional stages and when connecting to the soul the following phrases are held in mind before dropping them into the soul:

> May I live an authentic, heart and soulful life,
> may I live a life of ease and grace,
> may I be the best version of myself that I can be.

Exercise 6: Soulful Meditation script

'The first thing I would like you to do is to find somewhere quiet to sit for the next few minutes, get yourself into a really nice comfortable position sitting down, legs uncrossed, feet on the floor, rest your hands on your lap and if it feels comfortable close your eyes or if you prefer, just settle yourself on a neutral gazing spot in front of you.'

(Pause)

'Then start to bring your awareness to the movement of the breath into and out of your body............. notice how the air enters your nose into your lungs................ and then back out from your lungs through your nose into the room again............. Don't try to speed it up or slow it down, just allow it to be whatever it needs to be in this moment in time.'

(Pause)

'Allow the breath to anchor you in this moment.'

(Pause)

'Anytime those thoughts try and creep on in, just notice them and accept them and just allow them to pass on by............. bringing your awareness back to the movement of the breath into and out of your body.'

(Pause)

'When you are ready, bring your awareness to where you feel you connect with your soul and just rest there for a few moments. This may be a particular place in your body, all over or you may just be aware of the presence of your higher self, essence, a sense of "knowing" or "intuition" at a soul level. Don't try to force anything to happen, just allow yourself to connect with whatever comes up, holding in mind yourself at a soul level. You may then choose at a soul level to connect to a higher source whether it is the Divine Source, God, your own personal team of guides, teachers, helpers and angels. Make sure you set the intention to only ask

for support and guidance that comes from a loving, positive source which is for your highest good. Notice whether there is any discomfort or tension or perhaps a sense of calmness and peace. Just allow whatever to come up to come up without judgement or criticism, using your breath to breathe with your soul.'

(Pause)

'Connecting with your soul, bring up the phrases:

> May I live an authentic, heart and soulful life,
> may I live a life of ease and grace,
> may I be the best version of myself that I can be.

Imagine each of these phrases gently dropping into your soul. Be aware of whether there is any resistance or tension as you do this and using your breath, see whether you can embrace these sensations with loving kindness and acceptance.'

(Pause)

'Remaining connected to your soul, if you so choose, bring to mind a close friend or family member who has shown you unconditional love in your life. Notice any sensations that arise and just accept these as true to you in this moment, without censure or judgement.'

(Pause)

'When you are ready and feel connected to this person, offer them the following phrases:

> May you live an authentic, heart and soulful life,
> may you live a life of ease and grace,
> may you be the best version of yourself that you can be.

Imagine each of these phrases gently dropping into your soul. Be aware of whether there is any resistance or tension as you do this and using your breath see whether you can embrace these sensations with loving kindness and acceptance.'

(Pause)

'Still connected to your soul, and if you so choose, bring to mind someone who is neutral in your life. This maybe someone you notice when travelling to work, in the supermarket or when you are out walking. Just like you, they too may wish for a calm life, free from suffering and pain. Notice any sensations that arise as you bring this person to mind and just accept these as true to you in this moment, without censure or judgement.'

(Pause)

'When you are ready and feel connected to this person, offer them the following phrases:

May you live an authentic, heart and soulful life,
may you live a life of ease and grace,
may you be the best version of yourself that you can be.

Imagine each of these phrases gently dropping into your soul. Again, just be aware of whether there is any resistance or tension as you do this and using your breath, see whether you can embrace these sensations with loving kindness and acceptance.'

(Pause)

'Remaining connected to your soul, the next part is to bring to mind someone who has upset you or caused suffering or discomfort to you. Just like you, they too may wish for a calm life, free from suffering and pain. Notice any sensations that arise as you bring this person to mind and just accept these as true to you in this moment, without censure or judgement. If this is too difficult, then just bring your awareness back to your breath.'

(Pause)

'If you feel able to continue, when you are ready and feel connected to this person, offer them the following phrases:

May you live an authentic, heart and soulful life,
may you live a life of ease and grace,
may you be the best version of yourself that you can be.

Imagine each of these phrases gently dropping into your soul. Just be aware of whether there is any resistance or tension as you do this and using your breath, see whether you can embrace these sensations with loving kindness and acceptance.'

(Pause)

'Finally, connecting to your soul, and if you so choose, we are going to extend this Soulful Meditation as far as you feel able, to everyone in your street, home town, county, country, the entire planet, universe and creation. This can include all living creatures. Just like you, they too may wish for a calm life, free from suffering and pain. Notice any sensations that arise as you extend your mind as far as you feel able and just accept these as true to you in this moment, without censure or judgement.'

(Pause)

'When you are ready and feel connected to every living being and creatures that you wish to include, offer them the following phrases:

May you live an authentic, heart and soulful life,
may you live a life of ease and grace,
may you be the best version of yourself that you can be.

Imagine each of these phrases gently dropping into your soul. Again, just be aware of whether there is any resistance or tension as you do this and using your breath, see whether you can embrace these sensations with loving kindness and acceptance.'

(Pause)

'Now for a few minutes, bring your awareness back to your breath and the movement of the breath into and out of your body.'

(Pause)

'And then wherever you are with the movement of the breath, just start bringing your awareness to how your body is sitting on the chair, your feet resting on the floor, your hands resting on your lap. Notice the temperature of the air on your skin............ start wiggling your fingers and your toes............. and in your own time start opening up your eyes, bringing your awareness back into the room.'

Happiness versus grace

A key point to remind clients is that embracing a spiritual journey is an individual experience. It is important for our clients to be clear what their intention is from the outset. Do they want to have a deeper understanding of their life so far and the challenges they have experienced? Many people spend their lives striving or searching for happiness and view this as the answer to their difficulties. There are several books written to guide people in search of happiness, often by living a mindful life. However, Villoldo (2005) said that happiness is fleeting and casual and that grace, instead, is more transformative. He suggested that grace is achieved when the soul is completely healed from all past life wounds with the gained insight and wisdom from what caused the soul trauma. Grace enables us to be fully animated or awakened in life. Villoldo also said that 'in grace, you're free to be like the "lilies of the field" who need nothing, or those who "walk in the shadow of death and fear no evil", you just are.' To me, this represents authenticity, where a person lives a life of values and morals that are true to them and are based on pure unconditional love, rather than those that are ego-based or imposed by society or the environment. This doesn't always mean that they will be happy, but by living with authenticity and grace and learning self-love, they should feel more at peace within themselves.

Taking a leap of faith – becoming the driver not the passenger

There is no question that embracing a spiritual life usually involves some leaps of faith. It all comes down to whether your client continues to repeat patterns of behaviour and experience psychological distress and fear, or whether they want to be freer from discomfort, pain and suffering.

When clients take a leap of faith, it usually feels like they are jumping off a cliff edge without a parachute, not knowing whether they will land safely. It is learning to surrender to the fear that they have been holding on to that has been keeping them stuck repeating various life patterns or scenarios. Learning to make new choices and create a new template for their lives is exceptionally challenging at times, especially at the beginning of therapy and again, this is where encouragement and understanding of what your client is going through is imperative. Supporting clients in moving away from what is familiar to them can be frightening. Sometimes your client will feel a level of comfort with the familiar even if their experiences have been abusive or traumatic, feeling that it is easier when 'better the devil you know.'

Usually, these leaps of faith are there to show clients just that; when they take that leap, they have to have faith that it will turn out alright without knowing what the outcome will be, what will happen and what support will be provided along the way. If they knew all of this information beforehand it wouldn't be a leap of faith. The only thing that prevents them taking the leap will be their ego (or another's) convincing them that they are making a big mistake, highlighting all the things that could go wrong, telling them how they need to cling to everything in their life to survive. Learning to live a life through the heart and/or soul provides the foundation on which to base their leaps of faith. Whilst on their spiritual journey, clients will probably have opportunities to take several leaps of faith, perhaps in different areas of their life, for example, in work situations, in relationships and friendships. Helping your client to learn to recognise when these opportunities are being presented to them is part way there to taking that leap; the more aware and resourced they are, the more confident they will feel in taking that jump.

My own experience of living life through my heart and soul

Being on a spiritual journey can be quite subtle or rather intense. For me, it was subtle to begin with; growing up without the awareness and knowledge of how to really embrace the journey but knowing something didn't feel right in what I was observing. I learnt along the way as I went through life's challenges and experiences, and on many occasions, I was probably a slow learner as I lacked support or the skills necessary to help me break out of the ego cycle. I had many soul blocks and restrictions from this life and past lives that blocked me honouring my authenticity including: issues of judgement, criticism, inadequacy, sense of duty and responsibility, trying to fit in with others rather than respecting myself and so forth, and thus, I would often try and please others to my own detriment. Reflecting back, I can identify key moments when I was aware of the impact that both people and environmental situations were having on me at a heart and soul level. There have been many other occasions earlier in my life where I have been in situations where I did not feel comfortable; my body and whispers from my soul were telling me clearly when I was engaging in draining activities or when I was amongst people who were not necessarily nurturing my heart and soul. At times I would contemplate, 'I wonder whether if I got up and left would anyone notice or care?' For many years I did not honour these signs, I wasn't brave enough, listening to my ego that created the fear, scared of being judged or criticised for doing what was authentic to me and what the consequences would be if I did not conform to others' expectations or perceived judgements.

When I delved deep into soul level healing with the Akashic Records (discussed in more detail in Chapter 8) in 2016, I felt like I was in a washing machine on a full spin cycle with so much to purge and release from multiple lifetimes and this process continued at an intense pace for at least five years. I cried oceans of tears, and at times begged the universe for just a few minutes respite. After I slowed down the soul level healing and started to learn to trust my soul and the universe, opportunities to keep releasing and freeing myself from unauthentic situations and relationships continued. This meant I had to embrace some of my deepest fears, including people close to me nearly dying on several occasions. This involved directly experiencing a lack of support, significant failures and sometimes negligence in many different service care provisions. The world and parts of life that I was connected with seemed so broken. I had no choice but to completely surrender and cling to my faith, soul and the Divine. Any attempts to try and remedy the situation were met with more blocks. I also learnt to connect deeper within my soul when all other options felt extinguished and trust in my soul's journey for what I was here in this lifetime to experience. I was continuing to 'walk the walk' in order to 'talk the talk' which enabled me to support others when they later found themselves in similar situations of crisis.

Living life through your heart and soul – what to expect

During my life, I have had to face many deep fears. It has been a frightening and challenging journey and there have been times when I have questioned what I am doing and been close to giving up. I have also watched close friends go through a similar process and whilst it is natural for them to seek support and reassurance, and for me to provide them assistance, I have had to be careful not to become the rescuer and prevent them from getting to that deepest place themselves so that they can work through and integrate the learning and move forwards into their own authenticity.

The same is true for our clients. As therapists and clinicians we need to act from a place of compassionate support and understanding but not to act as rescuers. Rescuing others from their distress prevents them from learning that they are themselves strong enough to get through their difficulties. This fine balance may be difficult to achieve, but using a spiritual perspective, the more aware you become of why and how you respond in certain situations with your clients, the more informed you are of whether to act or hold back. If in doubt, ask yourself the question:

'What is my client meant to learn from this experience or situation to help them to move forwards?'

We can also ask ourselves:

'What am I meant to learn, teach or heal from supporting this client?' or,

'what is this experience teaching me?'

I emphasise and also warn clients that embarking on a mindful spiritual journey may alter their perception of life around them. The more aware they become of themselves and what feels true from a heart and soul perspective, the harder it can feel to fit into an everyday, 'normal' life. This isn't to deter anyone, but it is really important that clients are aware that their lives may change significantly, hopefully for the better, because they are becoming truer to themselves. It isn't unusual to find clients' friendships or interests change. Part of the process is letting go of all that no longer serves a purpose at a heart and soul level and instead learning to embrace that which nurtures them. This can happen quite subtly or very suddenly depending on circumstances and spiritual openness. The more authentic a life that your client can live, hopefully the less suffering and distress they should experience.

Summary

- The advantage of assisting clients to live an authentic life through their heart and soul is that it eases their psychological pain and suffering.
- Research studies have shown the benefits of working with clients at a heart to heart level where therapists spiritually resonate with their clients. Heartmath technology has shown positive physiological benefits of living life through the heart.
- Communications from the soul can present as opportunities to connect with the higher self and facilitate healing; it may occur in different forms of 'knowing' or intuition, ranging from visual, auditory, kinaesthetic, proprioceptive, and direct knowing.

- The Ful Trilogy is mindfulness, heartfulness and soulfulness. Learning to connect in all of these ways increases your clients' awareness of what their heart and soul are trying to communicate to them and enables them to start taking the journey towards living an authentic life.
- Making new choices that are heart and soul led may require your client to take leaps of faith. This can be an exceptionally challenging but rewarding process.

Chapter 7

Teaching clients HLP

'Whether one moves slowly or with speed, the one who is a seeker will be a finder.'

Rumi

This chapter will focus on how to teach your clients both the HL and HASL models of HLP which can be done as part of the preparation stages for EMDR therapy. I have provided scripts to help you explain the process to clients as well as a flowchart that you can follow, as illustrated in Figure 7.1. I would recommend that you start implementing HLP into your own life so that when you share this with clients you will have a deeper awareness and understanding of the process and be able to answer any related questions with authenticity.

Teaching clients the process of HLP

The HL model underpins both the HL and HASL models of HLP so I would start with this initially. If you have already had some conversations about spirituality during your assessment, you will have a sense of whether your client is open to the concept of a soul or not and this will guide you as to the terminology you use when going through the HL model.

To summarise, if:

- Your client is not interested or open to a spiritual perspective, or
- They are interested or open to a spiritual perspective but don't connect with the notion of a soul, or
- You haven't yet had an opportunity to explore spirituality with them then just use the word 'heart' when going through the HL model as this model is applicable to *anyone* regardless of their spirituality. If your client is open to the concept of a soul, then use the words 'heart and soul.'

HL script

I follow the description below to talk clients through the process, showing them a diagram of either the HL model (Figure 3.2) or HASL model

DOI: 10.4324/9781003509646-9

Is your client spiritual?

NO → Use Heart Led (HL) model.

YES → Use Heart and Soul Led (HASL) model.

Complete detailed assessment. Provide an HLP formulation to your client (based on challenges, traumas and significant relationships, blocks and restrictions, repeated themes that lead to psychological distress).

Explain about life lessons. Introduce HLP and the HL model diagram.

Explain about life lessons. Introduce HLP and the HASL model diagram. Discuss the idea of soul level blocks and restrictions and the option of soul therapies.

Teach client about the ego and ways to let go of the ego.

Teach client the process of becoming the observer.

HL model

Explore potential life lessons where clients connect with their heart.

Teach clients the value of making new HL choices and leaps of faith, identify the gifts and live a more authentic life.

HASL model

Explore potential life lessons where clients connect with their heart and soul.

Teach clients the value of making new HASL choices and leaps of faith, identify the gifts and live a more authentic life.

Encourage clients to use HLP with all challenges in their life.

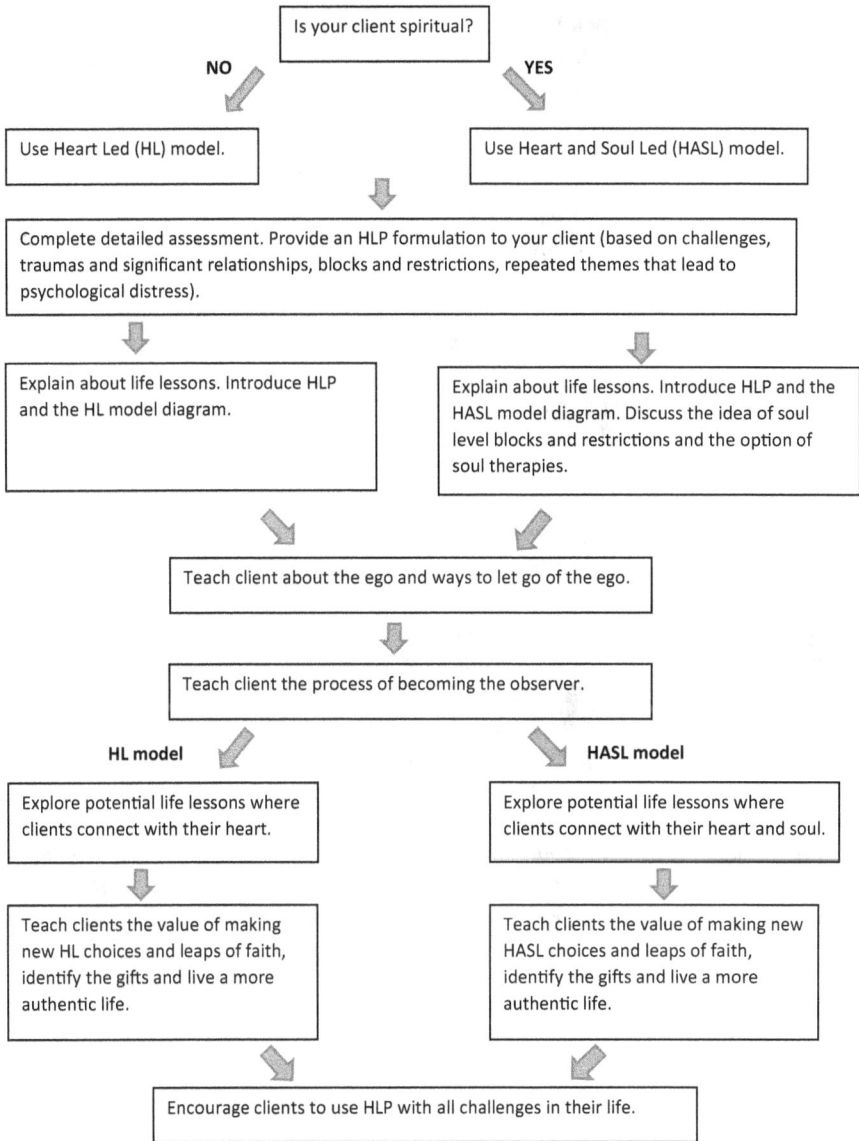

Figure 7.1 Flowchart of Heart Led Psychotherapy (HLP)
Source: © Alexandra Dent (2020). *Using Spirituality in Psychotherapy*, Routledge. Reproduced by permission of Taylor & Francis Group)

(Figure 3.3) at the relevant places where prompted. As I discuss HLP, I am always observing if it appears to resonate with them, noticing any changes in the energy levels with the client, either in the room or online, during our conversations.

Here is a simple way of teaching the HL model to clients:

'Life can be considered an individual journey in which we have opportunities to understand and experience life lessons. Life lessons are opportunities to learn, teach or heal others and ourselves. We all have our own individual primary life lesson and sometimes a few secondary life lessons, which are the key lessons we are trying to really understand throughout our lives. Examples of life lessons include abundance, empowerment, forgiveness, compassion and so forth. Life lessons are meant to be experienced in many different ways and in both positive and negative form. Take, for example, the theme of empowerment. This could be related to when to be empowered and when not to be so empowered, when to experience or not experience empowerment from others and so forth. Life lessons may effect just a few aspects of our life, or all areas, including: work, primary relationships, family, friends, hobbies, health and well-being, spirituality and our place in the community or our environment. We also may have joint lessons with a few significant people in our lives with whom we are working jointly to try and teach, learn or heal a particular theme. In addition, we have everyday life lessons that are opportunities to learn a wider range of attributes or themes to help us broaden and develop as individuals and to ultimately gain the most out of life. For example, you may go through a phase in life where many challenges are occurring in different areas of your life but have a similar theme, for example, assertiveness. Finally, there are the systemic life lessons that can be experienced where an event or trauma impacts at either a community, national or global level and this is another opportunity to work on additional themes beyond the primary and joint life lessons. It is important to keep remembering that we are all on individual journeys. It can be really tempting at times to try and help others but we have to remember that if we try and "rescue" others, even if our intentions are honourable, we are preventing them from learning their own lessons and this also diverts our attention from our own journey.*

We may all have had challenges in our life when we encounter difficult relationships with family members, friends or other people. This can make us believe that we are unlovable, that we don't deserve happiness, that we are to blame or that we are not good enough. We may also have found ourselves in difficult situations or traumatic experiences, possibly at school, in our neighbourhood, or in work, which could make us feel a failure, inadequate or powerless. All of these challenges can greatly effect us and when such difficulties occur and are not resolved, they become blocks and restrictions. Carrying these blocks and restrictions around with us makes it really hard when we have new challenges to face and we then often find ourselves repeating similar challenges and experiences throughout our lives.*

Although it can be very hard to recognise at the time, something positive can come from every difficult challenge that will enable us to understand the situation more clearly. A technique that can be used to break out of this repeated cycle is to learn to look at challenges with a different perspective and see them as opportunities to learn or experience something. This can change how we manage the difficulty and can help to lead to a more positive outcome. For example, if you have been in a difficult relationship, it may be an opportunity for you to learn to be empowered, or to have courage or strength, so that you don't allow someone to treat you again in a hurtful or abusive way. I would like to show you a model from a therapy called Heart Led Psychotherapy that provides a way of understanding challenges as opportunities to learn and experience life lessons.'

At this point I show the client the HL model and talk them through the stages *up until* the psychological distress, personalising to their situation and circumstances. I then introduce the topic of the ego (previously described in Chapter 4), as this is fundamental to the model. I am repeating the script again so that you can see how it fits in with the HLP process.

'There is a general acceptance that we all have an ego. The ego keeps us stuck in a repetitive cycle of repeated patterns of behaviour and maintains psychological distress. There is a general acceptance that we all have an ego. When I talk about the ego I am not referring to being narcissistic or self-righteous. Instead, I am referring to that part of us that creates our thoughts and desires and expectations. Our ego is very clever, it hooks us into people or situations because it makes us believe that we need these things in order to function or survive, but this creates dependency and we stop believing that we can function without such things. Our ego makes us both judge and feel judged or criticised, makes us take the blame for difficulties, or feel responsible for everyone else's happiness except our own. The problem is that when we live life through our ego, we often end up repeating patterns of behaviour or situations and this makes us feel stuck and trapped. We are never happy with what we already have because we are always searching for something else. Our ego doesn't want to be ignored so it provides very good arguments as to why we should stay stuck in challenging or difficult circumstances. Our ego creates FEAR about change, convincing us that something bad will happen if we make new choices – this is its biggest weapon.'

This is the stage where I explain about learning to become the observer.

'Life lessons are usually really difficult to experience and often we feel consumed by them and get caught up in the challenge. It is so easy to start feeling a victim to the experience, which makes us feel powerless and vulnerable, but it is our ego that is making us feel this way. Learning to step outside of the challenge and instead become the observer of challenges provides an opportunity to reflect on what is happening and helps us to view the situation differently with some detachment and heightened clarity. It helps us to start understanding

what the challenges are trying to teach us and to identify the life lesson so that we can make new choices instead of repeating similar themes or patterns in our lives that are ego-based. We become the victor rather than the victim which gives us strength and determination to tackle situations or people differently.

At this important stage we have a choice to make. We could make the same choices which come from our ego, but the difficulty with making ego choices is that they keep us stuck in the repeated patterns of behaviour and this maintains our distress and suffering. On the other hand, we can learn how to make new choices that feel right at a heart (and soul) level. Heart (and soul) led choices can be very hard to make and sometimes this requires us to take a leap of faith. This can feel frightening, as if we are jumping off a cliff edge without a parachute, not knowing whether we would land safely or not. However, if we knew the outcome it wouldn't be a leap of faith! When choices are made that honour our heart (and soul) rather than our ego, they are more likely to lead to positive outcomes and we can start to attain gifts; by this I mean a sense of gratitude, inspiration, freedom or truth and learn how to have self-love, self-belief, self-compassion, self-worth and self-acceptance. We then start living a more authentic life.'

Teaching clients how to implement key stages of HLP

Occasionally clients may already be practising the necessary techniques (discussed in Chapters 4, 5 and 6) to become more heart led and authentic. However, my experience so far is that the majority of individuals require extra guidance and support in this process. Some concepts may be familiar but clients struggle to implement them in their own circumstances. Many clients will say to me 'I don't know how to be in my heart' or 'I don't know what that means or what it involves.' The notion of self-love, self-worth and self-compassion is alien to them, maybe having spent their lives self-sacrificing, acting as rescuers or being martyrs. In these situations, I spend more time teaching them about the power of the ego, how to utilise mindfulness in their life and how to learn to move their awareness into their heart using the various exercises previously mentioned in the book, as well as additional techniques discussed below.

Becoming the observer, not the observed

This is a fundamental part of the model. It encourages clients to metaphorically step outside of the situation or challenge in which they find themselves, to view the situation as an observer and then, to reflect on what is actually happening in an objective way, without being caught up in the dynamics. Only at this point can your client begin to see this challenge as an opportunity to understand a particular life lesson. It is like asking your client to press the pause button on a film or a scene in a play, become the observer and start noticing what is happening with a degree of detachment. More often than not, when clients find themselves in challenges, they adopt the role of the victim, they feel hard done by and might feel someone else or the situation is punitive. They become so caught up in the drama or scene that they cannot reflect clearly as their distress is too overwhelming. Metaphorically stepping outside and being the observer allows the client to feel more removed from the situation and thus enables them to reflect with clarity and composure.

How to help your clients become the observer

1. Teaching Mindfulness

Mindfulness was discussed in detail in Chapter 5. Mindfulness is awareness, so the more mindful your client can become, the more aware they will be of recognising when they find themselves in challenges. This will then help them to follow the process of 'stepping outside' of the challenge and to observe, reflect, learn and take action. The quicker your client becomes aware of when they are snared in challenges, the quicker they will become the observer, learn lessons, make new choices and experience less suffering and distress.

2. Help Your Client to Recognise When They Are Identifying As a Victim

Difficult encounters with others or situations are typically very painful and challenging. This can make a person feel that they are the victim of others' behaviour or wrong-doing and, indeed, sometimes this is the case. The difficulty arises when the client's ego encourages the victim role long after the trauma, because it maintains the psychological distress. This is not a judgement or a criticism, merely a reflection of what typically happens. I myself have adopted this position many times in my life, sometimes, I could argue, justifiably but sometimes, perhaps not. Regardless of the circumstances, when your client identifies with the victim role, they feel a sense of powerlessness to change themselves or the situation and are not able to see clearly what they can learn from this experience. They become stuck and feel helpless. Learning to become the victor imbues your client with a sense of strength and power to look at what needs changing for their benefit and that of others so that they can make new choices and stop repeating themes.

3. Letting Go of Egoic Thinking

Several exercises to help clients to let go of their egoic thinking were provided in Chapter 4. Mindfulness will also make them much more aware of when their ego is present and having an impact on their distress. As you ask your client to take on the observer role, be aware of how they respond and whether observations are coming from their ego, heart or soul. If they are coming from their ego, help them to notice this with sensitivity; the ego can be clever and convincing and will put up resistance. Be patient and compassionate with your client as it may take them a while to learn to differentiate between their egoic thinking and their heart or soul messages.

4. Honouring the Heart and Soul

Encourage your client to learn to honour what their heart or soul is trying to communicate to them rather than their ego. You could use some of the exercises mentioned in Chapter 6. When your client honours what their heart or soul is communicating to them, they will be able to identify what they are to learn or experience from the challenges. This greater understanding will give them the ability to identify what new choices they can make.

When you teach your client how to become an observer, it is helpful to ask them to bring to mind a challenge they have experienced or are currently experiencing. I would then use the following script to show them how to become an observer to the challenge:

'I would like you to bring to mind that challenge that has been distressing for you. Imagine it is like being part of a play or drama where you are one of the actors in the play or drama. Once you have clearly connected with that challenge, imagine pressing the pause button to just stop or freeze what is happening. Now I would like you to metaphorically imagine yourself stepping out of the play or drama and become the observer.'

Once your client has become the observer, ask them the following relevant questions:

- 'What do you observe happening in this situation?'
- 'What do you notice happening between individuals in this situation?'
- 'What do you understand is the significance of certain individuals within this challenge?'
- 'Do you see yourself as a victim in this challenge and feel punished or hard done by?'
- 'What is your ego telling you about the situation or challenge that you are observing?'
- 'What is your heart (and soul) trying to communicate to you about the situation or challenge that you are observing?'
- 'How does it make you feel being the observer compared to being in the drama?'

Spend some time exploring their answers to the questions you have posed to them, again taking care to identify whether any observations appear to be ego-based, and if so, gently bring this to their awareness and see whether they can try to observe from their heart (and soul). This can take practice (for both you and your client) but remember the traits of the ego. If responses appear to be based on fear, expectations, hooks or the victim role, or any judgements or criticism, then it is highly likely to be an ego answer.

Life lessons

It has already been discussed in Chapter 3 that some spiritual views and beliefs propose the concept of life lessons. HLP utilises this concept, understanding life as being an individual journey in which there are opportunities to experience different life lessons. This concept can be used to provide a pathway to assist your client to express themselves with authenticity and self-love. As clients fully experience and understand their life lesson/s and work successfully on challenges and make the right choices, they may find that they are less likely to experience challenges with the same theme. If they get stuck, or continue to make egoic choices, they may find that certain challenges increase in order to help them with their understanding of their life lesson and enable them to make different choices that are heart and soul led. The critical point to remember is that as your client gains a level of knowledge and understanding about what they are meant to be experiencing it may ultimately enable them to make new choices and live a more authentic life.

Life lessons can effect your client in specific life areas or all aspects of their life. For example, they may effect work, finances, significant relationships, health, personal growth, spirituality, friendships, family, hobbies and interests or environment. Life lessons are not there because your client is being punished. Nor are they something that your client must achieve in order to 'learn' or 'grow' because they are lacking in some way. It is believed that the experience that clients can gain through the life lesson may enhance their ability to understand situations and themselves more fully and will guide them to make more informed choices that are heart and soul led rather than ego-led. In order to conceptualise life lessons and how they impact on your client, I have divided them into four headings; primary, joint, everyday and systemic life lessons. Again, this is based on certain spiritual beliefs rather than conclusive facts.

Primary life lessons

Your clients will have a primary life lesson and, possibly, one or a few secondary life lessons. They will encounter situations or challenges in order to help them experience these lessons so that they can be more authentic in how they choose to live their life. Life lessons tend to be extremely difficult and clients may have spent many, many, lifetimes working on these lessons, or they may just choose to experience a theme for a particular lifetime. Once a life lesson has been completed, the client no longer needs to have those experiences related to that life lesson; they have experienced them fully. It is not always essential to complete a life lesson; sometimes a soul will decide that they have gained enough understanding and that they do not need to continue with that particular lesson; they may decide to move onto something else, or focus on joint lessons and everyday life challenges. The critical point to remember is that as your client gains a level of knowledge and understanding about what they are meant to be experiencing, this will ultimately enable them to make new heart led choices.

Joint lessons

Most clients will have a few additional joint lessons, especially if another person is very significant in their life, for example, a family member or close friend. These joint lessons provide an opportunity to work on a slightly different theme to their primary life lesson in order to teach, learn or heal with another person. Joint lessons can be present just for this lifetime, or can be carried over from previous lifetimes if it is felt that the learning process is incomplete and further work in that area would be beneficial.

Joint lessons – being the 'rescuer'

It is not uncommon for clients to try and rescue others from their challenges and the associated learning as they do not like seeing others struggle or suffer. Whilst their intentions may be honourable, the problem with this is that this it comes from their ego, believing the other person needs their help, when in fact they are preventing the other person from learning and progressing for themselves; they are also not trusting that the other person's soul has knowledge, thus, implying that they know better. Sometimes, acting as a rescuer is a deflection and avoidance of having to face up to their own life lessons. The important thing to keep reminding your client is that they need to keep coming back to *themselves* and focus on their *individual* journey.

Everyday life lessons

In addition to your client's primary/secondary and joint lessons, they are likely to encounter everyday opportunities to experience different lessons. Interactions with other people, no matter how short in duration, are always opportunities to teach, learn or heal. Clients may notice a period of time in which there is a common theme to the issues or challenges they are experiencing; this will be occurring to broaden their understanding beyond their main life lessons.

Systemic life lessons

I have already discussed how life lessons can potentially effect us at an individual level. However, they may also impact on us at a systemic or global level and this provides another opportunity to understand and experience life lessons beyond the three categories already mentioned. Examples of systemic life lessons include: the numerous wars around the globe, natural disasters and various major tragedies including the September 11 attack on the Twin Towers in New York, 2001; the Manchester Arena bombing in 2017, or the racist murder of George Floyd in 2020 in Minneapolis. The global COVID-19 pandemic of 2020 is yet another example of the potential for systemic life lessons to be learnt. It provided opportunities for people to connect as a community, nation and internationally to offer support, kindness, love and change during adverse times.

Here are some of the potential themes for life lessons. This list is not exhaustive and I find that I add to it frequently while working with clients in this way:

- Abundance, acceptance, accountability, achievement, acknowledgement, appreciation, approval, assertiveness.
- Balance, beauty, blessing, bliss, boldness.
- Caring, centredness, charity, commitment, compassion, confidence, consciousness, consideration, contentment, cooperation, courage.
- Decisiveness, dependability, deserving, determination, discernment, Divine Love.
- Ease, empowerment, energy, enthusiasm.
- Faith, flexibility, forgiveness, fulfilment.
- Generosity, giving, grace, gratitude, growth.
- Happiness, harmony, healing, honesty, humility.
- Independence, inner authority, inspiration, integrity, intuition.
- Joy.
- Kindness, knowledge.
- Laughter, learning, light-heartedness, listening, love, loyalty.
- Mercy, mindfulness, moderation.
- Openness.
- Partnership, passion, patience, peace, perseverance, persistence, pleasure, possibility, power, practice, presence, protection.
- Receiving, recognition, reflection, reward.
- Safety, satisfaction, security, self-acceptance, self-assurance, self-belief, self-care, self-determination, self-love, self-worth, sensitivity, sincerity, spirituality, strength, success, surrender.
- Temperance, tenacity, trust, truth.
- Unconditionality, understanding.
- Vulnerability.
- Well-being, wisdom.

As already mentioned, themes can be experienced in both positive and negative form. Each theme therefore can have several messages to portray, and in different areas of a client's life and with different types of relationships, but all of these are important to allow the soul to fully express its true nature.

I suspect that I am not alone when I mention that 'receiving' is one of the everyday themes that I work on throughout my life. Most therapists and health care practitioners are very good at being there for others, they may be familiar with the archetype of 'rescuer' and perform acts of self-sacrifice but they do so usually at the expense of allowing themselves to receive unconditional love and support. When we start learning to be more heart led and authentic, it is important to be open to receiving unconditional kindness, support and love from others. I say 'unconditional' here because my experience early on in my life was that there were often conditions or guilt placed on receiving, even with the smallest things. This created an underlying belief that I was undeserving or unworthy of kindness and love or that I always had to give something back when I received, which created associated physical feelings of discomfort and unease. I am getting better at learning to say thank you and receive unconditionally, especially from trusted, beautiful friends so that I can surrender the belief that I have to be strong and do everything myself (this is a deep wound running through many, many lifetimes!). By learning to feel more comfortable with receiving, I am also allowing the other individual to enjoy the experience of giving. I am also learning when it is not safe to receive and have stronger protection and boundaries in place, especially when something is being projected in a harmful, abusive or unauthentic way.

When I am working with clients, I become curious as to what a client's life lesson/s could be. Table 7.1 provides some potential ideas that link recurrent themes or presenting issues with various life lessons. This table serves only as an example and is not definitive. Be curious and explore different possibilities as you see fit, based on your client's experiences and the difficulties they have had with making new choices. Remember, your client may be working on a number of different life lessons, including primary life lessons and possibly some secondary life lessons, joint lessons, everyday and systemic life lessons due to ongoing challenges.

Teaching clients to identify life lessons

Having helped your client to become an observer of their particular challenge, now is the opportunity to reflect and wonder together what their life lesson/s could be. As a therapist you are not meant to know the exact answer for them; usually your client will be able to give some ideas of what they think their lessons may be. This is how I introduce this stage:

'Now that you are the observer of this challenge or situation, what I would like you to consider, at a heart (and soul) level, is what this situation is trying to help you to understand or experience. What do you think the life lesson may be about?'

Some clients come up with ideas quite quickly. If they are struggling, use your intuition based on what you know about the client and their repeated themes and suggest potential ideas to see whether any resonate

Table 7.1 Potential ideas that link psychological issues with various life lessons

Presenting issue or recurrent theme	Life lesson
Depression, isolation, lack of joy	Empowerment; self-determination; courage, compassion, kindness, forgiveness, faith, trust, happiness, joy, strength, beauty, gratitude, bliss, laughter, blessing, appreciation, joy
Criticism, abuse	Truth, self-determination, assertiveness, self-worth, understanding, strength, safety, self-love
Being in unhappy or unrewarding situations	Self-belief, self-worth, autonomy, empowerment, achievement, recognition, inner-authority, approval, assertiveness, success
Trauma, loss	Forgiveness, compassion, courage, strength, self-belief, healing, Divine love
Acting for one's own needs and desires without recognising the impact on others	Integrity, courage, honour, honesty, truth, generosity, kindness, compassion, spirituality, humility, co-operation
Blaming others, victimisation	Mercy, Divine love, consciousness, accountability, understanding, humility, awareness, grace, empathy, acknowledgement, charity, wisdom
Destructive or unfulfilling relationships	Peace, harmony, partnership, forgiveness, compassion, strength, empowerment, self-worth, self-belief, possibility
Anxiety, worry, fear, doubt	Faith, trust, patience, ease, contentment, security, spirituality, safety, confidence, empowerment, strength, determination, surrender, acceptance
Misunderstanding, judgement, failure, self-sabotage	Compassion, clarity, self-belief, mercy, self-worth, deserving, understanding, giving, persistence, sensitivity
Obedience, timidity	Self-determination, self-worth, empowerment, courage, independence, co-operation, persistence, inspiration, receiving
Guilt, shame	Forgiveness, self-belief, self-worth, blessing, happiness, deserving, gratitude, compassion, pleasure, fulfilment, healing
Addictions	Moderation, tolerance, honesty, openness, deserving, faith, sincerity, abundance

with them at a heart (and soul) level. You could look at some of the ideas presented in Table 7.1 to act as a guide, whilst recognising that this table is not exhaustive and can be expanded upon as required. Sometimes a theme of a life lesson becomes more apparent over the course of a few sessions. Be mindful to work from the heart (and soul) and not the ego.

Identifying the gift

Each and every challenge, whether large or small, can provide a gift. This will usually be by truly experiencing and understanding a life lesson to enable the client to be more aligned to their authentic self and experience self-love. Initially, this idea can be particularly difficult for some people to conceptualise, because they are so caught up with being the victim that they fail to recognise that something good may come out of every situation. When life lessons are experienced and understood, new choices can be made to break out of the repeated themes that have previously been occurring and the pathway on the individual life journey becomes smoother. When new choices are made that are in keeping with what your clients' hearts and souls desire, rather than their ego, the gift is to experience more fulfilment, forgiveness, freedom and gratitude and live life with ease and grace rather than in turmoil and distress.

During particularly difficult challenges, it is likely that your client may need to take a leap of faith in a situation in order to achieve the gift. This occurs when clients understand a particular life lesson and are ready to make a new heart and soul led choice. Taking the leap of faith can be exceptionally challenging in itself and your client may experience extreme fear because the outcome is uncertain. However, once leaps of faith have been taken, your client will hopefully begin to feel relief and a sense of gratitude for their experiences regardless of how painful they have been. They may feel inspired and have courage and strength to make changes in their life that feel genuine and true to themselves when facing future challenges. Your client may notice feeling a sense of freedom, as they are no longer constrained by repeated themes, blocks and restrictions and they begin to learn to have self-love, self-compassion, self-belief, self-acceptance and self-worth.

Everyday life lessons and gifts

In my sessions with clients, I am increasingly noticing many opportunities to apply HLP to their everyday life challenges. If clients already have a good understanding of HLP and if I remain flexible with the structure of my sessions, we can explore everyday life challenges that have arisen between sessions, if appropriate. The benefits of this include helping them to gain increased awareness, empowerment and understanding about their challenges, as well as feeling more resourced to tackle further situations as they arise. Usually these conversations happen when events between sessions have occurred that make the client feel completely overwhelmed and exhausted. By reflecting on these challenges and applying HLP, clients often return to the next session reporting a sense of relief and freedom when they have managed to make new choices; this is part of the gifts they receive as a consequence of their actions.

Exploring the gifts gained and how to live more authentically

The following questions may be helpful when supporting your client to identify potential gifts:

- 'How can you use the acquired knowledge and understanding of your life lesson to take away something positive from the challenges you have experienced?'
- 'How can you apply this acquired knowledge and wisdom moving forwards when you encounter new challenges?'
- 'Are there any leaps of faith you may need to take to make heart and soul led choices and, if so, what would these be?'
- 'What coping strategies and resources do you need to support you in taking any leaps of faith?'
- 'Does making heart and soul led choices feel more authentic to you?'

Clients may need a great deal of support in this process. I cannot emphasise enough how hard it can be to make new heart and soul led choices and their ego may emerge many times to challenge them during this process. The more aware and prepared they are, the stronger and more able they will feel to manage this re-emergence of the ego. However, the benefits of living a more authentic life are so rewarding that this will give them strength to keep going. Living mindfully is a significant part of this journey and will help them to deal with the obstacles along the road and support them in stepping out of the Thought Bubble and egoic thinking. The more authentic you are as a therapist, the better the role model you will be to inspire and guide your clients.

Case example: Rose identifying the lessons and gifts

Rose was a woman in her early 30s with whom I had previously completed some EMDR therapy in relation to childhood sexual abuse and attachment difficulties. She contacted me four years later requesting a few further sessions because something sudden and traumatic had occurred and she needed some support in processing this. Rose was familiar with the ideas of HLP from our previous work and was actively practising regular self-care, including regular meditations and daily heart coherence using the HeartMath Inner Balance biofeedback system. We processed the latest trauma and the following session, Rose reported having identified one of her key life lessons through her heart-focused meditations which was 'empowerment.' She told me it was a relief to discover this and gave me a lovely example of practising being more empowered during a recent visit from her brother. He had been shouting and was being very angry and condescending about women. For the first time in her life, Rose stood up to her brother, asking him to stop shouting or he would have to leave. He continued so she asked her brother to go and Rose said she felt much more empowered as a result. Rose also mentioned that her beloved dog had suddenly died the week before. This was very sudden and unexpected as her dog was only four years old and had been fit and healthy. She told me she kept coming back into her heart during meditations and was shown the gift of self-forgiveness which she could generalise to many situations as an alternative to her usual egoic pattern of self-blame.

Additional components of the HASL model

Sometimes, simply using the HL model alone can empower clients to understand toxic, challenging relationships or situations differently, by following the process of becoming the observer in order to understand what the relationship or situation is trying to teach, learn or heal in themselves or the other person and make new choices so that the dynamics change. If, in spite of this, these relationships or situations continue to be challenging and your client is open to the presence of a soul and past lives/reincarnation, then it may be beneficial to consider the use of the HASL model (illustrated in Figure 3.3). The HASL model describes how potential soul level blocks and restrictions from past lives as well as current life may be impacting on their life and difficulties. It also includes the idea of soul therapies that may be a beneficial adjunction to the planned EMDR therapy. Soul therapies are believed by some spiritual practitioners to help identify, clear and heal blocks and restrictions at a soul level and this is discussed in more detail in Chapter 8. If you have started with just the HL model but at a later stage in therapy your client expresses curiosity about soul level or past life work, then you can always introduce the additional components in the HASL model.

Possible indications that soul level blocks and restrictions may be impacting on a client's life are where there are significant, toxic or enmeshed relationship difficulties. This could be with another key person (typically someone in their family, a close friend, acquaintance or work colleague), or it may be clear that your client has a major repeated issue with a certain aspect of their life, for example, finances, difficulty in conceiving children, or social, work or systemic issues. Even if a client may have some soul blocks and restrictions, this doesn't mean that they need to undertake soul therapies. Sometimes, just increasing your client's awareness of this area or teaching them some simple techniques to protect their energies (as discussed in Chapter 10) is enough to help them make new choices that are heart and soul led. More specialised soul level work with a suitable practitioner may be beneficial when a client wants to make changes but is really struggling, despite their best efforts. Clearing such blocks may help free them up and enable them to make the necessary new choices that are more authentic to them personally. Some EMDR therapists may have training in different soul level work or past life modalities and therefore feel comfortable including this in the package of care they offer their clients if clinically justified. For most, I would imagine that it is a topic you may raise with your clients, but then refer on to another practitioner who specialises in soul level work. Unless you are trained in offering soul therapies within your clinical practice, it is not your role to go into details with your client about what you believe may be their specific soul blocks and restrictions because you may well be wrong! Therefore, if you are even considering opening up this topic with your client, keep it as broad as possible, just open up the discussion that there may be soul blocks and restrictions and then advise your client to seek further support if they wish to discover more.

If your client is open to the presence of a soul, I would follow the same instructions as suggested in the HL script, using 'heart and soul' throughout. Once you have gone through this you can then introduce the idea of soul level blocks and restrictions. It is important to emphasise to clients that this is based on certain spiritual beliefs and not on scientific proof. I use the following description with my clients:

'There is a view that our souls are on a journey in order to learn a life lesson and that they go through many different lifetimes in order to facilitate this learning. What can happen during lifetimes is that we may have found ourselves in difficult or challenging situations where we have been forced to do something against our wishes. One example is being forced to marry someone we didn't love, often for the preservation of family honour, or not being allowed to marry someone we loved, because you, or your lover, were not deemed to come from a good enough or worthy background. We may have been forced to take part in a battle or fight in a war even though it was against our values. There are many different scenarios and this is what frequently happened in history – examples are plentiful in period novels and TV dramas, such as Pride and Prejudice. *When these situations happened and souls were forced to do something in conflict with their ideals, some believe that this created blocks and restrictions at a soul level. Ideas of such blocks and restrictions could include making vows of self-sacrifice, obedience, penitence, poverty or chastity. Sometimes contracts were made between souls, for example, a healing, protection or soulmate contract. Other potential blocks and restrictions include pacts, bindings and curses. The difficulty when such blocks and restrictions occurred is that they can be carried through to and impact on subsequent lifetimes. This can make it even more challenging to learn the life lessons and make the choices in keeping with our authentic self.'*

This is the point where I would present the HASL model to illustrate how past life challenges may lead to soul level blocks and restrictions that create repeated patterns of behaviour during past lives (see top left of the diagram). This then feeds into current life traumas which create current life blocks and restrictions. The other additional component of the HASL model is the option of undertaking soul therapy work to help clear soul level blocks and restrictions as discussed earlier.

Summary

- The aim of HLP is to provide clients with a technique to break out of the repetitive cycle that is maintaining their psychological distress.
- Clients are taught how to become the observer of their challenges so that they can assess the situation with a more detached perspective and thus identify their life lesson/s.
- Exploring the concept of life lessons can enable clients to make new, informed choices rather than repeating previous, familiar patterns of behaviour.
- Making new informed choices that are heart and soul led rather than ego led, encourages clients to honour their authentic selves and identify a gift from the challenge or trauma.
- Even if a client may feel they have some soul blocks and restrictions, this doesn't mean that they need to undertake soul therapies. Sometimes just increasing your client's awareness of this area is enough to help them intentionally make new choices that are heart and soul led.
- Soul therapies may be beneficial when a client wants to make changes but is really struggling, despite their best efforts, and it may be that the soul level blocks and restrictions are impacting on their ability to move forwards. Clearing such blocks may help free them up and enable them to make the necessary new choices that are more authentic to them.

Chapter 8

Soul level healing and Light Language

'Be soulful. Be kind. Be in love.'

Rumi

This chapter focuses on the area of soul level healing and how it can be incorporated into psychotherapy using the HASL model. There are now many different soul therapies available which are based on spiritual beliefs rather than scientific proof. Therefore it is impossible to prove the validity of such work. A few examples of soul therapies are discussed including the Akashic Records, shamanism and past life regression. Light Language, which is believed to be the most ancient as well as futuristic communication from the heart and soul, is then introduced and details provided of how this can be blended into all the different stages of EMDR therapy. If you are interested in exploring soul level healing for yourself or are considering discussing it with your clients, it is imperative that you do your own research and make sure you find a reputable and authentic practitioner. You may, of course, wish to or have already taken further training in various soul level healings, or know of colleagues who use these interventions. Work within your field of expertise and knowledge and always recommend that your client choose what resonates with them. If this is a new area to you, all I can encourage you to do is to try and keep an open mind and try not to form judgements or opinions based on ignorance.

The Akashic Records

The Akashic Records informs the key spiritual concepts underpinning HLP. The Hungarian philosopher, Ervin Laszlo, who was an advocate of quantum consciousness, described his belief that the Akashic Field represented an energy and information-carrying field that contained knowledge about all the universes past and present (Laszlo, 2007). Linda Howe (2010 p. 3) suggested that the Akashic Records is a 'dimension of consciousness that contains a vibrational record of every soul and its journey.' It is often referred to as a 'library' or 'Book of Life' residing in the 5th dimension (whereas we reside in

DOI: 10.4324/9781003509646-10

the 3rd dimension), containing every soul's pathway ever taken, including all past life memories, experiences, blocks and restrictions. O'Malley (2018) suggested that the eighth chakra (situated 20 cm above the head) can access the Akashic Records with the main functioning being to connect the physical body to a higher energy source.

It is believed by some (e.g., shamanic practitioners) that significant traumas, including emotional, physical, sexual or spiritual abuse, can cause soul level blocks and restrictions. Soul blocks can also be created or inflicted by various cultural traditions using witchcraft or black magic where there has been an underlying intention of causing harm to another. Examples of blocks include:

- Vows, e.g., self-sacrifice, obedience, penitence, chastity, poverty and suffering.
- Contracts, e.g., soulmate, healing and protection.
- Spells, curses, pacts and bindings.
- Anger spears and negative thought forms (in the Akashic Records these are believed to only happen in present life and are not carried through different incarnations).

We only have to look back in history to see how blocks such as curses, spells, vows and contracts were part of everyday life. Throughout the ages, individuals were frequently forced to participate in events that were against their authenticity, whether it be in war, marriage, work, religious or spiritual activities etc. The historian and author Philippa Gregory makes references to the use of enchantments, magic, spells and curses in some of her works of fiction (e.g., *The White Queen*). In certain areas of society and cultures today, there are still beliefs that cures, spells and black magic are used. Such blocks and restrictions may cause damage to:

- Chakras.
- Tears to the Golden Web which is believed to be an energetic membrane that surrounds an individual's energy bodies in order to keep the energetic being whole and integrated.
- God spark damage. It is thought that within our hearts there is an energy flame or spark that is representative of the Divine within us and is fed through an energy line that runs from the Divine Source.
- Soul facet loss, where part of the soul may have fragmented.

The process of the Akashic Record healing

An Akashic Reading usually provides information about one's soul profile, soul place of origination as well as one's main soul blocks and restrictions from either past or current incarnations. Once the Akashic Record clearing is complete, it is also possible to identify information about one's own primary and secondary life lessons as well as any potential joint lessons in subsequent sessions. A parent or carer can assist with clearing their children's Akashic Records on their behalf, up to the point at which their child becomes 18 years old. Generally, the child is unaware of this because they may not have the level of spiritually, insightfulness, or maturity to recognise the benefits of this work themselves. The child's soul will need to agree for this work to be completed, which is done by making a soul-to-soul connection and asking for permission.

It is imperative that any client embarking on this work consciously gives their permission for their Akashic Records to be read rather than feel they are being cajoled into undertaking this healing. It is believed that it is impossible to access someone's Akashic Records without their permission whether this is obtained consciously or at a soul level; the information will be blocked by their soul and the Divine Source. Therefore, it is trusting or having the faith that the soul must be in agreement and if it does not want to embark on this work, it will not occur. I have had personal experience of this where I paid for some healing for a friend who was going through significant challenges. At a 3D level, she was fully in agreement for this healing but when the practitioner came to do the work, my friend's soul blocked access to her Akashic Records. It was a lesson for me in trusting the process and also a reminder that whilst our intentions may be honourable, her soul was requiring that she still had to have certain experiences to learn important life lessons. She also needed to take the responsibility and ownership for her healing and individual journey.

I underwent a great deal of soul healing via the Akashic Records between 2016 and 2018. I was provided with detailed information about my soul and corresponding blocks and restrictions which were then cleared, a process overall taking around four hours each time. I was then given a customised 21-day prayer (which is very angelic and non-denominational) to enable the information to filter through to my everyday awareness and consciousness and confirming my intention for the healing and clearing. The next stage, integrating the healing and knowledge, is imperative. Whilst soul level blocks can be removed, it doesn't mean that such challenges won't happen again in the current lifetime. This is where the insight gained needs to be integrated. It is too easy to repeat familiar patterns of response and behaviour or stay stuck in situations or relationships, even though they may not be for one's highest good. The key part is to make different choices in life that are authentic to prevent such similar blocks arising again. Some people struggle with this phase, hoping that the healing will have done its magic and they don't need to do anything else. However, if they take this attitude, they are likely to re-create the blocks and fall back into repetitive patterns.

I completed Akashic Record training in 2017 which helped inform the key principles underlying HLP, but this is not a service I currently offer my clients. One of the reasons is that I like to maintain some professional boundaries, especially where clients have been referred via health insurance companies. I also believe that I am a catalyst for opening up the topic of spirituality with clients and that it is my role to guide and support them with the beginning part of this journey. I sometimes dowse client's life lessons in sessions using a pendulum if I have their and their soul's permission. Most of the time permission is granted but occasionally it is not. If not, I don't interpret this as an issue, and instead take the perspective that they are meant to determine this knowledge for themselves, or that the information isn't required in that given moment, but may be beneficial during a subsequent appointment.

As time progresses, different styles of practitioners are emerging who offer this service in a slimmed down version. There are also training programmes and books available to help individuals learn how to access their own Akashic Records. Sometimes, if a client feels there are soul level blocks between themselves and another individual that is causing them distress, I may suggest that they try to release any blocks by sending out an intention such as:

'I release all contracts, vows, curses, spells, bindings, hooks, anger spears, negative thought forms or any other block and restriction between myself and this person all the way back to point of origin in my Akashic Records.'

Ask your client to connect with their heart and soul as they do this, to ensure that it is coming from a place of love. I would encourage them to do this as often as they feel necessary to deepen the intention into their consciousness. It is important that they also consciously attempt to make heart led choices moving forwards with that individual, allowing the learning to be integrated.

I have worked with some very good practitioners but unfortunately have also had some bad experiences too (where the practitioner may have an inflated ego, charge a lot of money and not work authentically) so using discernment is imperative if you are interested in participating in such work.

Shamanism and soul retrieval

A number of psychotherapists have incorporated soul retrieval and shamanic journeying into their practice, for example, Alberto Villoldo (2005) and Sandra Ingerman (2014) who describe Shamanism as a pathway to opening up and learning to live life through one's heart, ideas in keeping with HLP.

Shamanic journeying typically involves the use of rhythm, often through drumming, as this is believed to help individuals enter an altered state of consciousness so that they connect with the spiritual dimension of reality. The word shaman comes from the Siberian Tungusic word for a spiritual leader or 'one who is raised' and this title can often be interchanged with medicine man/woman or healer. Shamans believe that there are three worlds: the Middle World, which is where we physically exist, work and have relationships, and the Lower and Upper Worlds, which are not physical places, but archetypal and energetic realms that are not bound by time. The Lower

World is the realm of the soul and contains all information on our soul's history, in other words, our past. The Upper World is the realm of our destiny and our spirit and energetically travelling to this world can help access our destiny and life purpose. It is believed that, working with an experienced Shaman, a person can enter the Lower and Upper Worlds to discover information that may assist them in making sense of their lives. Travelling to the Lower World can also help retrieve missing parts of their soul that may have been lost through past traumas. As mentioned earlier in the book, Irene Siegel (2017, 2018) integrates aspects of shamanism into her EMDR sessions.

Past life regression

The aim of past life regression therapy is to heal mental, physical and spiritual issues by identifying, reliving and resolving past traumas. It is based on the belief that past life traumas are held in our etheric, mental and physical energy fields (Tomlinson, 2012). These traumas may have occurred in this lifetime or past lifetimes. The process typically involves using hypnosis to guide the client into an altered state of consciousness so that they can 'bridge back' and reconnect with the original trauma. Once connected, clients can gain a greater understanding of what the situation was that caused the trauma and find ways to process and heal the trauma. Often this involves forgiveness, either to the person who caused the trauma, or perhaps to the recipient of the trauma.

Other spiritual healing techniques

There are many alternative or spiritual therapies continually becoming available depending on one's own belief system including Angelic Reiki, traditional Reiki, working with crystals, chakra clearing, yoga, various types of massage, acupuncture, reflexology, herbalism and homeopathy to name but a few. I have met a number of alternative practitioners who work at a past-life level, including reflexologists, acupuncturists and homeopaths. If your clients are interested in alternative therapies, the key is that they find someone they can trust, because, as with any type of practitioner, some are wonderful and incredibly talented and others may not be so authentic.

Karma

Discussing karma is controversial. Many of us prefer to avoid the concept of karma, let alone discuss what it could represent or mean to us. When we think of the idea of karma, most people assume they have done something terribly wrong to explain their suffering or discomfort. For example, if a person has an illness or condition, or finds themselves in tough circumstances, they may blame this on 'karma.' I personally do not feel this view is not a fair representation of karma and it can lead to confusion and misunderstandings.

Different religions and belief systems have various interpretations of karma which of course makes the whole topic very confusing. The Sanskrit interpretation of karma is based on action, work or deed, as well as cause and effect, where the intentions of an individual (cause) have a bearing on the future of that individual (effect). It distinguishes between good and bad karma. If someone has performed good deeds in their life this will result in good karma. On the other hand, if an individual has had the intent of causing bad or harmful deeds in life then this will lead to future suffering. Tomlinson (2012) explained karma as a way of experiencing both sides of a situation and how this may be carried over various lifetimes to facilitate greater understanding and development.

From an Akashic Record perspective, Howe (2010) recommends not to view reincarnation as 'good' or 'bad,' or karma in terms of 'reward' or 'punishment.' In Akashic Record training, karma is differentiated between 'negative unjustified karma' and 'negative karma.' It is believed that negative unjustified karma occurs during a situation where a soul has been forced to do something against their wishes, or that goes against their Divine purpose. In contrast, negative karma is believed to occur between two or more souls. If someone has consciously killed, or been instrumental in the death of another individual, then it is believed that this creates negative karma at a soul level because this action goes against the Divine Source. Therefore, the soul who was instrumental in someone else's death would be considered the 'bearer' of the karma and the soul who died would be the 'recipient' of the karma. In subsequent reincarnations, the bearer and recipient souls may enter into another situation or relationship to provide an opportunity for the negative karma to be healed. The way to heal negative karma and break the pattern is to learn to approach the situation differently. This requires the 'recipient' to operate with an open, loving and compassionate heart and show forgiveness to the 'bearer,' whilst also teaching them through love and compassion to take responsibility for their wrongdoing.

Negative karma is the only block or restriction that cannot be cleared using the Akashic Records. In a similar way to how Tomlinson (2012) described using past life regression, it is believed that the only way negative karma can be cleared is for the recipient to teach or heal the bearer about true forgiveness, and support them in aligning with a more positive loving way of living through unconditional love. Negative karmic relationships are very challenging and may present themselves in abusive or toxic relationships. The difficulty is that the soul bearer of the negative karma usually lacks the insight that they have done anything wrong and tends to blame the soul of the recipient for any difficulties. The recipient typically encounters abusive or destructive behaviour from the bearer and often becomes the victim over and over again. Thus, these relationships end up in vicious, repeated patterns of behaviour. Negative karma can be healed when the recipient learns to step outside the fearful victim role and take a different approach. This usually involves the recipient putting up protective boundaries while keeping their heart and soul open with divine unconditional love, forgiving the bearer and holding on to the intention that the bearer may become a kinder, more loving and compassionate person.

With all soul level work, it is important to not become too attached to the information gained because this in itself can create the victim role, clinging on to the trauma, rather than processing the trauma and integrating the lesson; 'I was hung or burnt at the stake in a past life' or 'this person forced me into a loveless marriage or took my children away.' Encourage your client to be connected in their heart to allow forgiveness, compassion and love in the eternal, ever-present moment.

Light Language

Light Language is considered by some to be the most ancient form of communication of the heart and soul as well as a futuristic communication. It is believed to work at an energetically high vibration and frequency, connecting with the cosmos, Divine, different realms and multidimensions. It is also timeless, so one can listen to it several months or years later, and still gain benefit. It can be expressed through different methods including words, drawings, tones, movement and perhaps even more ways we have not yet discovered.

Light Language can often be considered analogous to speaking in tongues. From my perspective, speaking in tongues appears to have its history within a religious context and is referred to in the Bible. To me, Light Language does not need to be bound up in a religion or religious practice, it is a spiritual experience, connecting with a divine, unconditional source of love. In other words, Light Language may be experienced by a wider group of people than speaking in tongues – but there is no reason to say that speaking in tongues is not an aspect of Light Language. Religious people may consider themselves as spiritual but spiritual people are do not necessarily consider themselves religious.

Everyone has the potential to communicate Light Language, it can lie dormant in our energy field and be activated either by another person, place or situation at various stages during one's spiritual or healing journey. I am aware of some EMDR therapists who channel Light Language although not necessarily in their EMDR sessions. Light Language is not something that you learn through a traditional teaching style, it is a channelled healing. The key is to stay out of the ego and not analyse, judge or interpret what is happening. The ability to use Light Language also doesn't mean you are 'special' in any way, but it is important to recognise that it is a spiritual gift that needs to be used wisely and with authentic purpose.

Since 2023, Light Language healing has gone viral on social media platforms and whilst I feel there are some amazing Light Language healers around the world, there are also those that are less authentic or pertaining to offer 'powerful' healing to potentially very vulnerable individuals. There is a huge variety in how Light Language can sound, be seen or felt depending on who is delivering it. If you are interested in experiencing this healing then please do tune into the authenticity of the person and check that it resonates. I have listened or watched some individuals and feel absolutely nothing, or at worse, feel their inauthenticity. However, there are others where my body or energy field did feel a connection.

I had never heard of Light Language before November 2018. While taking part in a spiritual retreat in Glastonbury, UK, I heard a guest musician speak Light Language in combination with his music. It really resonated and touched my soul. In January 2019, a colleague sent me a link to an American woman who spoke about the sacred heart and professed to be a Light Language activator amongst other things. I felt drawn to have some online healing sessions with her and with time started speaking a few words, but was blocked by my ego, which created doubt, judgement, fear and embarrassment. Initially, I was anxious about speaking it with other individuals so I practised speaking to trees and in nature to build up my confidence. This progressed over the year to speaking some Light Language to close friends, and then by 2020 I had started to integrate it into my clinical work, including EMDR sessions. I received very positive feedback from clients and I have since presented Light Language at various transpersonal psychology and EMDR conferences and trainings. When preparing a webinar for the EMDR Association in 2024 on using spirituality in EMDR, I showed a colleague a video of an EMDR session where I had used Light Language with a client. I was asking for some advice as to whether it was suitable, acknowledging my own anxiety and vulnerability about showing something that may be perceived as unusual or controversial. After playing the ten-minute clip, my colleague reflected back a sense of surprise and curiosity about how the Light Language had just impacted on her personally. She said: 'I felt my heart rate decreased. I was feeling stressed, headachy and it just helped calm me and feel like I had some space in my head.'

This was consistent with feedback from my clients and friends who also reported feeling calmer after hearing my Light Language. One possible explanation for this, purely based on qualitative feedback I have received, is that the Light Language may be helping to calm a person's nervous system as well as supporting them to connect to their heart, although I appreciate I have no current scientific evidence to back this up.

Using Light Language in EMDR therapy

I never plan to use Light Language in sessions. I could go for weeks without using it at all and then notice times where I am using it with most clients. I have not yet managed to see any correlation as to when Light Language flows through more; it does not seem to be dependent on my own energy levels or astrological events but it does come in bursts. It's a spontaneous channelling and can take me by surprise at times, especially when in the middle of an EMDR processing session. The Light Language I channel tends to be around two to five minutes long each time which fits perfectly with an average length of time of BLS sets. Light Language has come through at all stages of EMDR therapy, from the initial assessment phase, preparation and resource work, desensitisation phase all the way through to completion. I have used it alongside various energy techniques, for example, I channelled some Light Language with one client who was using the protection and clearing resource (described in Chapter 10) to remove some of the negative projections she was feeling from her narcissistic ex-husband. At the end she said: 'that was incredible and really powerful. I now feel I can handle him and the situation.'

I once had an EMDR colleague tell me that her client began to speak in tongues during the processing. I have also had a handful of clients who were already able to speak Light Language and they started channelling this during their EMDR processing sessions. However, at the moment, I would suggest that this is unusual, but with time, may become a more frequent occurrence. If your client does start speaking Light Language or in tongues during EMDR processing, just allow it to flow, and do not intervene or start asking any questions. You can always have a short debrief at the end of the session. I have sometimes recorded some personalised Light Language for my clients which they can listen to in between sessions to add to their own resource box.

So far, I have not received negative feedback after speaking Light Language with clients. Even the most sceptical people are able to express a sense of curiosity and openness. If I sense some Light Language wanting to come through during processing, I will wait until I have had feedback from a BLS set, and then briefly introduce Light Language, always obtaining permission before speaking it during subsequent BLS sets. My intention is to keep the flow of EMDR processing as smooth as possible, avoiding any long discussions, which can be reserved for the end of the session if needed. I usually introduce Light Language by saying:

'I'm just wondering how you would feel about me sending you some healing during the next set of processing.'

If the client gives you permission, then I will say:

'There's some healing that I offer which is called Light Language. It's my heart and soul connecting with your heart and soul and channelling some unconditional divine love. I am not sure if you have watched the film series The Lord of the Rings, *but the Light Language I speak sounds a little bit like how the elves communicate with each other. You are unlikely to be able to make any sense of it at a conscious level, but your heart and soul will understand and receive the messages required. I will just be speaking Light Language quietly in the background whilst you continue the EMDR processing.'*

Usually, the client is curious at this stage, but I will instruct them to reconnect with what came up during their last BLS set before starting the next BLS. I will then channel the Light Language for as long as it comes through, often in the form of words but also movement of my hands. I continue with the desensitisation processing as per the standard protocol, stopping when appropriate to ask what the client is noticing, making sure of course that I allow enough time to end the session properly. In some sessions, a lot of Light Language may come through, especially if I sense some negative energies or soul level blocks and restrictions require assistance to be cleared. Sometimes, if the client is abreacting, then Light Language comes through to assist them through this process. Each client and session are a different experience and my job is to step out of the way and trust the process, allowing whatever needs to come through to come through. I rarely try to interpret what is happening or to suggest ideas to the client as that is not my role. My job is to facilitate the processing and allow the Light Language to flow without too much interpretation or analysis.

Whilst it may feel that new and advanced healing modalities are on the increase, most could be considered to be ancient forms of wisdom, teachings and techniques that stem back to the origin of time. This wisdom may be deeply embodied in our souls' DNA and energy fields, carried through many, many lifetimes, and is only re-activated at various times in one's soul journey when the soul and physical body are ready to connect with and apply this knowledge. Such energy and wisdom can be used for good or bad purposes. Powerful healing techniques have sometimes been abused when not in alignment with the Divine, hence the use of curses, spells, bindings, contracts and black magic. I have had a few clients who mention that they feel they are quite powerful spiritually, but sense that this is not always done in a positive way, which can frighten them. If this is the case, it is very important that they are supported to be more heart-centred and aligned with the Divine or a loving essence that resonates with them. It may be that they have had past lives where they feel they have abused their spiritual gifts and these past lives would benefit from clearing and healing so that they can integrate the learning and start making new heart led choices moving forwards in their journey.

Summary

- The Akashic Records are believed to hold all the information of a soul's journey throughout its lifetimes and contains the knowledge of all life blocks and restrictions at a soul level.
- Clearing soul blocks and restrictions can facilitate your client in making new choices at a soul level rather than repeating recurrent themes. However, this is now a conscious choice on how to live their life; they may still decide to repeat themes even though the blocks and restrictions have been removed.

- It is believed that negative karma is the only block that cannot be cleared using the Akashic Records or past life therapies. The importance of negative karma is that resolution and forgiveness is achieved during a lifetime between the souls concerned in order to heal the negative karma.
- Light Language is considered by some to be the most ancient form of communication as well as futuristic.
- Light Language is an example of a healing modality can be incorporated into EMDR therapy at all stages in the process to assist with multi-dimensional and soul level healing.

Spiritually informed EMDR therapy

Chapter 9

EMDR Phase I

History-taking

'The wound is the place where the light enters you.'

Rumi

Part 3 of the book focuses on integrating spirituality and HLP into each of the eight phases of EMDR therapy. This chapter focuses on phase 1 of EMDR therapy which is the history-taking phase. The importance of observing the energetic connection with your clients from the moment they make contact with you is emphasised, holding on to this awareness throughout the duration of working with your client. The key areas to cover during a detailed history are discussed, including how to integrate HLP as part of a BioPsychoSocioSpiritual approach to treating trauma. Ideas of how to explore the topic of spirituality and energy with clients are presented, along with case examples, to illustrate the variety of responses that can be obtained. Guidance on what to do if your client is not spiritual is also explained. Lastly, formulating using a BioPsychoSocioSpiritual approach and HLP perspective is covered and illustrated using a working case example.

A BioPsychoSocioSpiritual approach to history-taking

Observing the energetic connection

When a client makes initial contact, I am aware that an energetic connection has already begun and how I instinctively take an 'energetic' reading of the situation. I am also aware of the transference and countertransference process. I observe how I feel or respond to that initial connection and try to establish whether I am meant to get involved or not, investigating any resistance I may feel, whilst also trying to surrender and trust the spiritual process that the clients I am meant to work with will find their way to me and act as my mirrors and teachers too. When I meet the client for the first time, whether in person or online, I have a level of curiosity about how they settle into the energetic space that I have prepared and how my energy changes in their presence. If several individuals arrive, for example, couples, parents/carers and children, I observe the energetic connection between them as well as myself.

DOI: 10.4324/9781003509646-12

I set the intention to form a heart-based, Divine connection with the client, aware that at this stage, they are often unable to sense or feel the true Divine light within themselves. I seem to be developing an internal, energetic radar that detects energies that may be carried in the client's energetic system that does not belong to them, but may be impacting on their wellbeing. Sometimes these energies may feel very dense or heavy but I rarely mention it at this stage and if I do, I am very careful how I convey this information; this may be more appropriate when I am offering a formulation which would include a spiritual or energetic perspective, having asked them if they feel they have absorbed other people's energies whilst growing up or in various relationships throughout their life. I hold a level of curiosity about how my energy changes during various parts of the session and in reference to what is being discussed. Often, if I notice my energies feel scattered, this is an indication to me that the client is not very grounded or may be quite dissociative, so it is important to do a few grounding techniques (discussed in Chapter 10) to settle the client within themselves so they can get the most out of the session. The more you work with energies with others and within yourself, you are likely to find you become more heightened and sensitive to noticing subtle changes, especially if you have undertaken various healing or soul level trainings, or regularly utilise spiritual practices such as Qi Gong, meditation or reiki.

During my core therapy training, the importance of taking a detailed history was really drilled into me. I equate this to searching for all the pieces of a jigsaw puzzle, putting this together to make sense of what has happened throughout the client's life. This enables me to provide them with a clear formulation, check that it resonates with them and then devise a suitable treatment plan, taking into account their goals, which are re-evaluated during the treatment process. It might sound obvious, but I am aware through supervising other EMDR therapists that some professions adopt less rigorous approaches when taking an initial assessment.

Another advantage of completing a detailed background history is that it allows the key areas within HLP to be explored. As discussed in Chapter 3, some spiritual concepts believe that relationships formed, with work colleagues, neighbours, friends, acquaintances or someone we meet for a brief time, provide an opportunity to *teach, learn and/or heal* (both ways). When relationships are very challenging, this may indicate potential blocks and restrictions from current or previous past life encounters at a soul level (Weiss & Weiss, 2012). Throughout the assessment process, I am holding the HLP model in mind. I am looking for evidence of:

- Challenges, traumas and attachment/relationship difficulties.
- Current/past life blocks and restrictions.
- Current/past life repeated themes.
- Possible life lessons (individual, joint etc.).

Background history

The assessment may take several sessions depending on the client's experiences and complexity of attachment history and trauma. Whilst I hold a semi-structured framework in mind about areas that I need to cover, sometimes the client just needs to offload in that first appointment and we will focus on the background history next time. I believe that the most important aspect of the initial assessment is to establish and build an energetically safe, trusting and containing therapeutic connection and relationship. This is my priority and I work very hard to establish this from the outset because without this very little will be achieved. I make no assumptions at this stage that we will work together, as I need to make sure we can create an energetic fit and resonance. I let clients know that I am aware they are checking me out to see if they can work with me, and I also tell them that I am also establishing whether I am the best person for them too. If not, then I will support them in finding someone suitable for their particular needs.

Current issues

After welcoming the client, settling them into the therapeutic space (whether online or in person), and having completed all the paperwork and confidentiality agreement, some initial questions I might explore include:

- What current issues are they struggling with that has brought them into therapy at this point in their life?
- How are these current issues impacting them in their daily life?
- How would they describe current relationships in different areas of their life, including family, friends, school or work colleagues, neighbours or peers?
- What has initiated their desire to seek help now?

Genogram and family history

I then begin to take a detailed family background history. I always complete a genogram (a graphic representation of a family tree) of significant family members, including parents, grandparents, aunts and uncles, siblings and children. This is highly informative, as it enables me to explore the dynamics and relationships with and between family members, as well as determine who may also have experienced medical or psychological difficulties. During this process, I am looking for any history of suicide, psychological breakdown, ancestral, inter-generational and cultural trauma.

I then explore the relationships the client has had with significant key people in their life (both positive and negative), including within their family, neighbours, teachers, friends or within their wider community. This may include spiritual, religious or cultural groups, organisations, or institutions that they have or currently belong to which may or may not resonate with their own personal identity. Who showed them love, nurturance, care, compassion, acceptance, safety and containment, and how was this communicated to them; was it verbally and physically or mostly through behaviours?

When you start assessing from this perspective, you begin to recognise patterns quickly, highlighting:

- Possible primary or joint lessons that might be playing out between different family members or the wider community.
- Who at a soul level may be representing the teachers, learners or healers in the family or the wider community.
- Potential soul or ancestral blocks and restrictions, such as vows of obedience, suffering, poverty, contracts, negative thought forms, unjustified or justified karma.
- Themes such as disempowerment, self-sacrificing, victimisation and addiction.

Sometimes a client may report having overheard or directly experienced people saying that they were unwanted, or that they are responsible for all the family's damage and hurt from a very young age. I have had some clients become consciously aware of these projections as early as in utero during EMDR processing. I am curious about both the positive and negative movement in energy, that may take the format of beliefs, emotions and behaviours between family members or the wider system/community. For example, there may be family members (or individuals within the wider community) who gaslight (mislead or manipulate with intention) and who are unable to take any ownership or responsibility for their actions and behaviours. Often you will see these patterns continuing down through the generations, but one or two members of the family or community may be the more 'energetically sensitive' and awake members and attempt to break free from these cycles. Clients may have chosen to incarnate to heal their own as well as generational, ancestral or cultural wounds, but in doing so, have ended up being the punchbag for the projections from others. These clients may feel ostracised or segregated by their family or community for believing that something isn't quite right, or for not engaging in similar behaviours. They are likely to have learnt to dissociate from an early age as a survival mechanism, due to the overwhelming projections and trauma experienced. Identifying potential key moments when this happened can provide possible targets for EMDR processing.

Dobo (2023) discussed how predominantly using two main core negative cognitions 'I am not good enough' and 'I don't matter' (which can of course contain many other cognitions within) transformed his EMDR practice. Other negative cognitions that I have frequently observed when working spiritually with EMDR clients include:

- I don't fit in.
- I am different.
- I am not important.
- I am bad, unworthy.
- It's my fault/I am responsible.
- I am unlovable.
- I am not safe (in one or many areas, e.g., physically, emotionally, spiritually, cognitively).

Developmental and educational history

The next stage is to explore the client's developmental and educational history, keeping note of any absences or lapses in their memory which could indicate dissociation. I am keen to know what their experience was like during their education and school years and whether there is a history of any form of trauma, perhaps from bullying, discrimination, marginalisation or oppression. I am curious as to when they first noticed any psychological issues, such as anxiety or depression, and what triggered these. Do they have a history of self-harm, suicidal ideation, alcohol, smoking, drug or psychedelic substance use? Have they ever received any therapeutic support, and if so, what was their experience of this like, or did their distress go unnoticed?

Depending on the age of the client, I then explore what working opportunities they have had; have they been able to maintain a job, work relationships, career, or has this been variable and inconsistent? All the way through this, I am trying to identify possible blocks or negative beliefs that are creating repeated patterns/cycles in their life. Have they experienced discrimination, marginalisation or oppression in any area of their working life? From an EMDR perspective, I am constantly looking out for traumas and significant events that may signify unprocessed material, noticing how the client and their energy levels react to discussing various areas of their life; do they become tearful or withdrawn, unemotional or resistant to discussing any area?

Identifying blocks and restrictions and repeated themes

Repeated themes are often indicators of blocks and restrictions, including intergenerational, ancestral, cultural, societal, etc. that have occurred, for example:

- Do they constantly find themselves in very destructive relationships, groups, situations or environments?
- Did they ever receive love or positivity through their early life experiences, relationships, communities or environment and if not, what impact has this had on subsequent relationships?
- Do they feel trapped in relationships, groups or situations that are draining but cannot find a way to make changes?

- Do they struggle to believe they can have happiness, peace, faith or trust in others or themselves?
- Does their underlying negative beliefs impact on the choices they are making in their life?
- Are they constantly self-sacrificing and not getting their needs met?
- Is money, health, love or relationships a repeated issue, either believing they are not worthy, or struggling to hold on to something when it is going well?
- Do they self-sabotage situations?

If an individual has had very difficult early attachment relationships, one of the repeated themes they may experience is struggling to have intimate or emotionally close relationships with others. They may instead remain detached, because positive relationships and emotions are unfamiliar and frightening to them. This is likely to impact on any future attachments where they may remain emotionally numb, anxious or depressed. Sometimes such clients may meet future partners, friends or members of a community where certain individuals represent the role of a teacher or healer and are trying to show the client love and nurturance. The key area here is whether the client is able to internalise and experience this positive relationship. For example, I see adult clients who experienced very poor attachment relationships in early life and have learnt to shut down and dissociate from their emotional responses as a survival strategy, which creates blocks and restrictions. They meet someone who is able to offer them love, and provide a nurturing and supportive relationship, but more often than not, they still find it immensely difficult to open up and receive love and affection from others. They may continue to believe that they are worthless, undeserving, not good enough and unlovable. Despite managing to maintain a relationship with someone, their ability to accept the positive emotions from others can still be impaired. On this level they are still stuck in the repeated themes or repeated patterns of behaviour.

Another indicator of clients having repeated themes is when they present in a resistant or emotionally detached manner in the therapeutic relationship. Their protective wall is there to keep them safe, so trying to engage in a session will probably make them feel uncomfortable and frightened. Just being in a session with you could make your client feel outside their emotional window of tolerance, especially if you are engaging them with compassion and kindness. If this happens, I give them an understanding as to why they feel this, so that they can learn to understand rather than see this as a problem. I explain that part of my work is to help them to feel more comfortable and with time, they can learn to integrate the positive effect of our therapeutic relationship.

Identifying positive relationships and resources

During the process of identifying repeated themes, it is also important to try and find any positive situations where your client has made new choices that have resulted in a change of direction from earlier repeated themes. I take note of any positive relationships throughout their life where they have managed to break out of a familiar pattern to form more healthy, supportive connections either directly with another person or maybe within a group or community setting. At a soul level, whom did they bring into this incarnation that are supportive figures, and at what stage in their life did this happen? This could be resourced if required in the preparation stages of EMDR. I am also identifying any nurturing, wise, and protective figures which can be installed later on. Such resources may then provide great spiritual assets or interweaves during EMDR desensitisation. Even though a person may be really struggling in life and feeling very isolated, knowing that they have a spiritual support team that they can access regularly can be hugely beneficial and provide strength and courage.

Some positive areas to explore, if you feel your client has made new choices, include:

- What facilitated the new choice? Was it a new partner, another significant individual, situation, group or community, or a change in social setting or circumstance?
- Were the new choices made from their heart and soul and more in line with their authentic selves?
- To what extent did making a new choice result in a different outcome?

With practice, noticing repeated themes and patterns of behaviour gets easier and easier. The greater the depth of spiritual understanding of the therapist, the stronger their intuition and the more rapidly they can become aware of such repeated themes and patterns of their clients.

Additional components

Towards the end of the assessment, I inquire about their current sleep and eating patterns, any prescribed medication, current suicidal ideation (if present), what activities and hobbies they are participating in, what social support they have available to them and also what are their goals for therapy. I may ask the client to complete some questionnaires to assess for dissociation, mood, anxiety and trauma, spirituality and mindfulness. There is currently not a massive choice of suitable questionnaires available to explore mindfulness and spirituality but two that I have used include the Mindfulness Attention and Awareness Scale (MAAS), (Brown & Ryan, 2003) and the Inventory of Secular/Spiritual Wakefulness WAKE-19 (Kilrea et al., 2023). Some clients find a few of the questions hard to answer or make sense of so it is always sensible to go through and support them in this process. Mbazzi et al. (2021) reported that questionnaires are not routinely used within African populations as they tend not to be culturally appropriate or understood.

Goals

Finally, but importantly, I ask what the client's goals are if they haven't specified these already. I want to make sure these are achievable and realistic and that I have the skills to support them.

Exploring spirituality with your client

The topic of spirituality may arise during any of the stages of the EMDR process or it may never happen at all. Sometimes, your client may open up about their spiritual beliefs or experiences quite spontaneously from the beginning. They may want to focus on this during the first session, especially if they are aware that this is an area you specialise in, and have sought to connect with you for this very reason. If this is the case, then allow it to happen, knowing that during further sessions you will still need to cover the background history in order to obtain a good understanding of their life, especially if you are going to move on to EMDR processing.

Sometimes there may be small indicators of a spiritual openness, and it may feel appropriate to ask about their understanding or belief system, whether it is spiritual or related to the idea of energies. On other occasions we complete the background history and I will open up this topic at the end. Rarely do I not explore this with clients nowadays, but there are always some clients to whom it doesn't feel relevant or appropriate, so I try to keep in mind whether it is clinically justified or not. Be guided by your client and only explore spiritual concepts that they are familiar, comfortable with or have expressed an interest in understanding further.

Divine energy can be used both positively and also destructively and abusively. Sometimes, a client acknowledges that they engaged in bullying or punitive behaviour to others as a way of dealing with their own traumas. They may show some awareness and concern that they feel have a level of power to influence or harm others and have not always used this with good intent. This may indicate areas for processing, and I have had a few clients who felt this could be related to past life experiences. My job is not to prove or judge this, but to support the client with the meaning that it has for them and be aware that during EMDR processing, past life material may surface that can help them make sense of this and heal any associated wounds or trauma.

Spirituality is often experienced as a deeply personal and private connection between an individual and the cosmos. Clients can be vulnerable in many areas of their life, including spiritually, and it is imperative that we aim not to take advantage of this by forcing or inflicting our ideas or beliefs onto them. You can use any of the questions discussed in Chapter 2 where you explored your own relationship with spirituality, but be careful not to overdo this with clients. Always consider what is the rationale behind asking questions and are they pertinent to the work that you may feel will benefit them rather than asking just for the sake of asking. Adopting Socratic questioning keeps the dialogue open and curious. A simple and effective question to start the process of enquiry is usually:

'I was wondering what your spiritual beliefs are?'

It is perfectly acceptable to ask them to elaborate further if you are uncertain about what they have said, for example:

'Please could you tell me what you mean?' or

'I am not familiar with that but I am really keen to learn, please could you tell me more?'

This may open up an informative and significant discussion about their spiritual beliefs or experiences, and at the very least, it will do no harm. If they respond by saying:

'I am an atheist, I don't believe in a God and don't care what happens to me when I die,'

then this is probably a good time to move on to the next part of your session. It is however, important to acknowledge their views as true to them and it is not your role to try and convince them otherwise. A simple response may be:

'Thank you for sharing, that is really helpful to know.'

This does not mean that you cannot use the ideas and concepts of HLP at various stages during therapy, because the Heart Led (HL) model is applicable to everyone.

Sometimes a client responds by telling you which particular religion they belong to, and this may lead on to a discussion about what their belief system or experience has been in relation to this. Robin Shapiro (2009) provided three groups of questions which are more of a religious-spiritual nature to explore with clients which include asking about whether the client has been raised in a particular religion or faith tradition, what connection they have with that religion or faith currently and whether the family's tradition was common in the area where they grew up. It is also important to identify whether your client may have experienced spiritual abuse.

When exploring spirituality, you can always use the questions offered in Chapter 2 which can be applied, adapted and elaborated depending on how your client responds. Attune to the feedback you are receiving both in the transference and any subtle or overt shifts in the energy of the session as you have these discussions, because that in itself is useful information. Depending on how the discussion is progressing, and if the client has expressed interest in spirituality, I usually ask whether they believe in the presence of a soul. This allows me to take the conversation slightly deeper, and provides an indication as to the depth of therapeutic work possible. A simple question to ask is:

'Do you believe that we have a soul?'

A person's answer to this can be very informative. If they answer *'yes'* or *'maybe,'* then I will ask:

'What do you think happens to the soul when a person dies?'

The client may have never considered this idea but express some openness or curiosity and if so, then I may follow up by asking:

'Are you open to the idea of past lives and reincarnation?'

Remember that how a client responds will inform you of whether you can use the HL or HASL model. If you do not know much about a particular spiritual area or religion that the client is discussing then it is advisable to find some time to research this, and there is plenty of information and literature easily accessible now online, in books, etc. Try to hold a level of discernment, curiosity and a non-judgemental attitude to what you discover and if something gets triggered within yourself, be open to explore what this represents to you outside of sessions, so that this does not impact too much on the transference, countertransference and energetic resonance during your sessions. However, don't be afraid to say to the client that your knowledge is limited, but that you are keen to understand more and hear about their experiences, always being curious with what the meaning is to them.

I used to get feedback from clients saying that they were surprised a 'psychologist' would be open to a spiritual approach, expressing how important it was for them to be asked such questions, especially if it is, or has been, a significant part of their life. They feel able to integrate spirituality into their therapeutic work, feeling a sense of relief and keen to take their healing to a deeper level. It is not uncommon for clients to tell me that they used to have spiritual experiences when younger, but that these became repressed because they were not around people or in an environment that understood or supported such concepts. In this way, I am acting as a catalyst to reignite this within themselves. As with the other areas explored during the history-taking, I am noticing the energetic changes that happen during different parts of our session and how these relate to the topics we are covering. How does the energy or vibration with the client, within myself and in the room shift as they share their spiritual experiences?

It is understandable for an individual to question at times their own spiritual or religious beliefs, especially in the context of great suffering or trauma, whether this is something they have experienced personally or is happening at a global level. They may be questioning the meaning of such trauma or looking for someone or something to blame, or somewhere to vent their anger. This can be especially challenging when a person has experienced spiritual abuse, which adds further confusion, especially when it is in conflict with their belief system.

A few examples are provided by Shapiro (2009, p. 486) who suggested that the loss of one's faith may be more traumatic than the event that led to it. Care and sensitivity are needed when discussing such areas. It is not our role to minimise, justify or judge but to provide an empathic, accepting and curious approach whilst keeping an awareness of when something is triggered in us to explore safely with our own support system outside of the session.

You may find that some clients actively seek a therapist who is not from their particular religious or spiritual background. This might happen if the client is concerned about seeing someone from their own cultural background or belief system who might then judge them, their behaviour, or be unable to provide a safe space to question or explore their beliefs.

Exploring 'energies' with your client

Whether clients are open to spirituality or not, I usually explore the concept of energy, whether they are aware of their own energies or emotions, and how these change when in different situations or relationships. The word 'spirituality' can be triggering for some depending on their background and can also get easily confused or entangled with the idea of religion, yet 'energy' is much more neutral and accessible. Energies were explored in more detail in Chapter 2.

A nice way to ask this is as follows:

'I wonder whether you are aware of how your energy changes when you are in different situations or with different people? For example:

- Do you feel drained or depleted if you are near someone who is feeling angry, sad or anxious?
- Do you feel uplifted and energised if you are with someone who is in a positive and joyous mood?
- Are there certain places or situations where you notice your energy or mood changes, e.g., in a work situation, a certain environment or physical location such as when you spend time in nature, a city or a busy environment?'

Usually, a client can relate to the above scenarios recognising the impact that other people's energy or situations have on them, but tend not to be very good at protecting their energy, especially when the experience is negative. I have also noticed that sensitive people, and those who have had early attachment issues or trauma have learnt to soak up and absorb the difficult emotions from those around them as they grow up. This can saturate their energy field with dense, low vibrating energies. Perhaps, at a heart or soul level they believe that this will help their situation or those people around them, but the problem with this is that it is often to their own detriment. A frequent comment that clients with early attachment trauma reflect to me when we explore the concept of energies is 'I had to learn to read the room from a very young age.' By this, of course, they are referring to sensing the energy of the room, detecting if it was safe enough to be 'present,' because early life trauma had heightened their sympathetic nervous system responses and they had learnt to scan for danger.

I have found discussing energies to be such a useful part of the history-taking process because it helps provide information about what protective resources may need to be learnt, what can be installed as positive resources during the preparation stages, as well as potential areas to target during EMDR processing. Areas to consider exploring include:

- Does the client seem to be absorbing other people's energies at the expense of their own or feel they are being drained by others?
- Do they know how to look after and protect their own energy system using suitable energetic boundaries?
- Who are the people with whom or places where an individual feels calmer or safer that enables their nervous system to be regulated?
- What are the triggers that cause distress that could be areas for processing?

It would be highly unusual to offend anyone by asking about their spirituality or energies unless you start to impose your views or your client feels you are judging or mocking them. I believe that as time goes on, there is more acceptance and openness to this topic. It is increasingly my experience that it can play a significant part in people's lives and that not asking the question closes down a whole area of work that could be extremely powerful and helpful for the individual.

Common themes to be aware of during the history-taking process of the energetically, highly sensitive person include, but are not exclusive to:

- Difficulty fitting into their surroundings and society.
- Loneliness.
- Trust issues.
- Difficulty forming close relationships and friendships.
- Feeling misunderstood.
- Gynaecological difficulties.
- Gastrointestinal difficulties.
- Sexual or intimacy difficulties.
- Sensitivities to sounds, smells, sensations.

As I am sure you will see, there is such an overlap of these themes with many current diagnoses, but when taking a more informed spiritual history-taking, we are also applying an energetic lens and considering this within our formulating using a BioPsychoSocioSpiritual approach.

Questions about spirituality and energies: client examples

Below are some of the responses I have received over the past few years in response to asking about clients' spiritual views or beliefs. They come from a variety of ages, sexual orientation, socio-economic backgrounds, cultures, etc.:

- I believe in God. I was brought up a Catholic. Goodness comes through people. I believe in a soul but only in this life. I hope the soul has peace and no suffering when the body dies. Scotland holds a lot of happy memories for me, nature is soothing as are animals.
- I would consider myself quite a spiritual person and open-minded. I believe in a soul that is on a journey and also believe in past lives. We can have a soul purpose and can become unhealthy if not in alignment. I also believe in a greater energy which is more nature-based (Mother Earth, Gaia).
- I belong to a Sikh family which focuses more on being a human and a better person than religion. Sikhs are always learners, open minded. I want to find self-love. In respect to the soul, I feel such characteristics stay within the family.
- I have a saying that comes to me every year, for example, 'control the controllable,' 'matching energies.' I believe in manifestation as well as a soul and can feel other peoples' souls. My Nan was the same, intuitive. I am open to the idea of reincarnation and other possibilities although unsure what this looks like.
- I believe in something, more so with energies. I don't have a view on death but I believe in an essence.
- I haven't thought about it much. I was brought up as a Catholic in Ireland. I have been in a relationship with a Muslim who would like to talk about his beliefs. I believe in a soul which is an inner goodness. I am not sure about after life. I take my mother to church regularly.
- I am a Christian and love to be open. I believe there is more to the world than we understand. I believe in star signs, and sound therapy but have not had a network of friends to support this. I love the idea of being spiritual. I believe in a soul and feel my grandmother looks over me.
- I believe in things that are scientifically proven. Also, that you can influence your own energy. I do not believe in spirits or shamanism but do believe in the idea of energy. I believe in a soul but that it dies when the body does, so do not believe in reincarnation.
- I don't have any but I wish I did to help think what I am going through is for a reason. I recognise the idea of energies and how my energy changes when I am with certain people or in certain situations.
- I am an atheist. I feel a connection to nature, animals and water. I can get sentimentally attached to things. I kept a brick for years, and feel a strong connection to buildings. I don't believe in a soul but do believe in energy. I feel drawn to things when people are not around.

- I would not consider myself as religious. I believe in a masculine and feminine god that is all loving and always there for you. Everything has a lesson and something valuable for you. I don't have any specific thoughts on life after death or past lives but can feel the presence of those that I knew who have died.
- I meditate and believe in chakras. I love nature, everyone has a soul or an entity. I believe we are here for a reason to learn lessons and believe in reincarnation. I believe in star seeds and manifesting. I am a Christian, believe in God, and feel we are all connected. I get déjà vu feelings. People come in to your life at the most ridiculous times, even the ones who hurt, so you can learn something. I experience a lot of serendipitous moments. I am not really connected to the idea of past lives.

As you can see from the examples provided there is a huge variety in responses, with most resonating with either the idea of a soul, an essence or the idea of energies.

What if you, or your clients, are not spiritual?

Not every client will be open to working spiritually and that is fine. What I have observed is that whilst some people may not resonate with the word 'spirituality,' when I use the word 'energies,' virtually everyone relates to this. This may then become our chosen common language, enabling clients to learn to protect and understand themselves as an energetic being. The key concepts from the HL model can also still be discussed as a general framework, without any reference to spirituality, and integrated into the therapeutic work. This can provide some wisdom along the way, and guide people to not only understand how to handle everyday life challenges, but also how they can learn and grow from opportunities. Many people now seem to be keen to make changes to their life to break out of familiar and stuck patterns or cycles, and make different choices that are in alignment with their authenticity.

Formulation

Once you have completed your initial assessment, you will be in a position to share your formulation. The formulation can include a spiritual or energetic perspective. I have given an example in Chapter 11 of a general narrative formulation that I sometimes read to those clients with difficult early attachment histories, either at the end of the history-taking phase, or as part of the preparation phase.

The formulation can incorporate a HLP perspective to your EMDR formulation. This would reflect how your client's current psychological distress may be based on the challenges and traumas, blocks and restrictions and repeated themes or cycles they have experienced that remain unprocessed, and held in the non-adaptive state. I remain curious about what client's potential life lessons may be, especially the primary and joint life lessons, how much of their difficulties have resulted from living an ego led life and what different heart led choices and leaps of faith may be required to assist them to move forwards. I take into account how their experiences and relationships have impacted them on an energetic and spiritual level as well as how much other individuals' energies could have been absorbed over their lifetime, which may still be affecting them currently.

Treatment plan

In terms of the treatment plan, I assess how insightful and motivated the client appears to be at making different choices and what resources and intervention are required to facilitate this to meet their goals. I only discuss EMDR therapy at this stage if I am absolutely sure that the client has the ability to self-soothe, is able to develop a therapeutic relationship with me, has some form of connection with the outside world, is not highly dissociative or at high risk and is committed to change. EMDR is a very powerful and transformative therapy and I need to trust that the client is willing to engage with this work. They need to be made aware that as they start to align with their heart and authentic self, they may be confronted with opportunities to take leaps of faith, including making significant changes to various relationships and situations that they have been stuck in for many years. Their outlook on the world and their perceptions will change. Therefore, obtaining informed consent from your clients to carry out this work is advisable. The treatment plan is kept under regular review and amended and adapted accordingly throughout the therapeutic process.

For those clients with much more complex histories and trauma, the treatment plan may be more open and include psychoeducation, mindfulness and other resource work, HLP, ego state and inner child work with the potential to complete trauma-based work at a later stage. Whilst EMDR therapists know that EMDR is an 8-phase model and this may be explained as such, most clients only view phase 4, the desensitisation phase, as actually having received EMDR therapy. In my experience, it is safer and kinder not to create too many expectations for the client, especially if they need a lot more preparation and stabilisation, otherwise they may believe that they 'have failed or are not good enough to be able to do the processing phase of EMDR.' When I feel confident that the client has engaged and is progressing well, I will take the opportunity to explain about EMDR in more detail. The exception to this would be if you provide intensive EMDR therapy where significant support and containment is available for your clients.

Case example: Javid

Background history, formulation and treatment plan

Javid was an Iranian-born man in his 40s. He attended sessions at the request of his line manager, who had observed Javid not being himself, easily agitated, emotionally charged and moody. Javid had started work enthusiastically with his current employer at the beginning of the COVID-19 pandemic in 2020 but he had found the first few years quite isolating. Javid was struggling with various aspects of his work and the constant complaints from his stakeholders and colleagues were getting him down. He reported feeling emotionally drained, dreading work, overthinking and procrastinating and was working weekends to catch up with his tasks. He reported being easily triggered by seeing couples argue and mentioned having regular nightmares and flashbacks. Most areas of his life were quite isolating. He described himself as an introvert, not happy with his current living arrangements and had a limited social network, spending most of his time at the gym, running or hiking. He didn't have a good eating routine and frequently drank alcohol in the evenings. Most of his family resided in Iran. He was at the point of resigning when I met him and was fairly unconvinced about the benefit of attending therapy sessions. He admitted that he was sceptical of therapy as he felt it would require a lot of work and he was unsure whether he was prepared to commit to this. Ironically, he also reported reading a lot of self-care books as he was seeking answers to why he struggled, suggesting he had a level of awareness that something needed to change.

The background history was completed over several sessions. My main focus was on engagement and connecting in an energetic, containing and safe way with Javid as he was very unsure about committing to therapy. During the second session, I learnt about his upbringing. Javid told me that he had grown up in a war zone, and half of the children in his neighbourhood didn't survive beyond the age of 20 years old. He had little recollection of life before six years old. His parents lived in different locations for significant amounts of time during his childhood. His paternal grandmother had looked after him and his siblings between the ages of six to 12 years old, after which his parents moved back with them all. He described being loved and nurtured by his paternal grandmother, although she was also strict. His mother was on a lot of medication for various health-related ailments and he was not aware of any major issues with her or other family members, but admitted that he wouldn't know, as this was never discussed. He also mentioned having witnessed something very traumatic when he was eight years old that he could not speak about, but was still impacting on him significantly. When his parents moved back when he was 12 years old, Javid described this as "horrible." His father was strict and religious and they would be woken at 5 am to do prayers. He described his father as physically violent to everyone and emotionally unavailable.

Javid's parents had lived apart for the past 22 years, and he told me that he had not been on good terms with his father, as they didn't see eye to eye. He didn't feel close to his mother, but had respect for her for what she endured during her marriage. He was only in regular touch with one of his two brothers who was residing in China.

Javid was a very bright man. As a child he was top of his class in primary school and was seen as a 'role model' by his teachers. He struggled during middle school, where he reported failing more and being isolated, but he managed to re-apply himself during high school years. He had always had a passion to fly, but the government had strict rules about what careers were available to people from different locations and origins, and this was not an option for him. He underwent compulsory military service for two years, which he struggled with. He felt discipline was used without due course and this continued to give him nightmares. However, he described this time as also liberating as it was his first time away from his family. He returned to the family home and tried to support the family business, but this wasn't a positive experience, so he tried various jobs before taking employment with an English company in Tehran. He moved to the UK when he was in his mid-30s and also completed further educational courses including Masters courses, most of which he self-funded, at the same time as trying to financially support members of his family back in Iran. He had various employments, some of which involved global travelling, before settling in his current role. He mentioned having a few short-term relationships, but only one in which he lived with a European lady for a year. During this time, he reported feeling suffocated and was aware of the age and cultural differences, especially from her family, who were concerned he was going to kidnap her and take her to Iran, and made threats to report Javid to the police. This relationship felt especially sad because it felt like he was being judged unfairly because of his culture. This also made him anxious about entering new relationships in case something similar occurred. In his daily life, Javid reported observing other people and constantly questioned, "what is wrong with me?" When discussing HLP, I still recall Javid saying "the concept of living through my heart is alien to me," thus highlighting how much of his life and experiences had been dominated by ego thinking with little space for him to embrace his authenticity. Even the few chances he had attempted to do this, for example, his desire to become a pilot after school, were prevented by his government. Javid was open to the idea of a source of unconditional divine love or energy. He described his spiritual views as:

"I grew up a Muslim, my father was very religious. I practised this until my late teens, and when I started military service, I stopped asking myself why I was doing it. I believe in good and bad. When I moved to the UK, I felt like religion was a façade and didn't believe in it, it was indoctrinated into me as I grew up and I have dismissed 95 per cent of this. I would like to leave the world a better place and I enjoy contributing to charities. I don't believe in God. I believe that what goes around, comes around. Honesty and integrity are very important to me. I believe in a soul although unsure what happens to it when we die and I am unsure about reincarnation. I am more spiritual than materialistic."'

Javid's goals included:

- Something needing to change in him to be happier in life.
- Become less triggered by small things.
- Feel calmer and peaceful for longer periods of time.

At the end of the second appointment, I provided an initial HLP-informed for-mulation based on his attachment difficulties and trauma experiences. Javid's challenges, traumas and attachment issues included:

- Poor attachment to both parents and complex family dynamics, including a violent father and mother with health issues (intergenerational trauma).
- Growing up in a war zone (cultural trauma).
- Significant trauma at the age of eight that he was unable to speak about, but was still impacting on him significantly.
- School bullying.
- Academic challenges during middle school.
- Some traumas when attending military service.

Javid's underlying blocks and restrictions were:

- High expectations of himself, very self-critical and judgemental of self.
- Sense of being a failure, not good enough, unlovable, unworthy and not feeling safe.
- Sense of financial responsibility for supporting his mother and family back in Iran.
- Having soaked up or absorbed other people's projections, beliefs, emo-tions, traumas and energies from all areas during his life.

Javid's repeated themes appeared to be:

- Sense of loss throughout his life especially in relationships (whether through war, family dynamics or cultural issues).
- Avoidance of forming meaningful relationships.
- Keeping himself isolated and having a small social support network.
- Minimal self-care.
- Cultural issues and not feeling able or safe to integrate or fit into different societies.
- Feeling unsettled, unfulfilled with jobs and accommodation/environment.

Javid's possible life lessons included self-worth, empowerment and self-belief. His father also appeared to be a key person in his life, with a possible joint lesson between them.

Formulation

*I helped Javid to understand that when a baby or small person experiences dis-
comfort or distress, they rely on their parents or significant adults to attune to
their needs to help them feel safe, soothed and contained, perhaps by being cud-
dled, rocked to sleep, fed or changing nappies. This enables the small person to
manage their discomfort and feel safe. However, when Javid was a baby and then
a small boy, he didn't have many key adults in his life that had the resources and
tools to help him manage his discomfort or distress. Perhaps this was because
they hadn't experienced or been shown this when they were themselves little, so
had never had healthy role models. His mother had her own health issues, his
father was aggressive, and the family were living in a very dangerous environment, suggesting his sympathetic nervous system had learnt to become very activated and always on alert. Javid may have also absorbed many difficult emotions
and beliefs from his environment, not only having lived in a frightening war zone,
but also from key family members, as well as possible ancestral and cultural
trauma. We discussed how Javid would have had to learn how to manage these
difficult feelings from a very young age, possibly using dissociation to block out
the discomfort and help him survive. It was likely that he was still dissociative,
even though his circumstances had changed, which was making it hard to have
meaningful positive, healthy relationships. I explored with Javid, using the HL
model, how his early life traumas and challenges had created various blocks,
restrictions and underlying core NCs, including a sense of failure, being unlovable, unworthy, unsafe and not feeling not good enough. These appeared to be
maintaining repeated cycles in different areas of his life. I explained the impact
that his ego may be having on the choices he was making which was resulting in
him experiencing ongoing psychological distress.*

Treatment plan

*From the start, I could sense so much light and potential within Javid, but he
was unable to recognise this within himself. My initial focus and treatment plan
was just to calmly hold the energy of unconditional hope and light, and see
whether Javid was able to attend sessions and engage therapeutically. I also
focused on teaching him resources from the start, which included him watching
the three online workshops (psychoeducation of trauma, mindfulness and
HLP), learning affirmations and installing a peaceful place. I also taught him
other techniques to help him take more care of his energies, so that he could
start noticing an improvement in his overall wellbeing, as well as preparing him
for EMDR. Whilst initially slightly cynical about therapy, Javid embraced all
the resources, and started applying what he was learning to his current life.
Before starting EMDR processing, his heart-based affirmations were already
starting to manifest; he secured a new role within his organisation, which gave
him the opportunity to work abroad for three months, which he relished.*

Key memories we identified and targeted included domestic violence between parents growing up, living in a war zone, a sense of failing during middle school and undertaking military service. We initially targeted the domestic violence between his parents and school-related issues and Javid was amazed at how quickly some of the images faded, but he took longer to release the many physical sensations and emotions held within his body. At times, we used the two handed interweave (Shapiro, 2005), *and on one occasion when it was hard for him to release anger, he found a safe place to release this, by imagining himself floating in the ocean. During some of the EMDR sessions, Javid was able to recognise that he was carrying other people's energies within his own energetic field, which he managed to clear, allowing me to assist with Light Language. Javid found EMDR a very positive experience and was able to apply heart and energy interweaves to facilitate the processing. It was during the processing of the unspeakable trauma, aged eight years old, that his primary life lesson became more apparent. The theme was forgiveness, and with time Javid was able to start forgiving those who had been involved in that trauma, as well as himself for having witnessed the event. He was then able to apply this to other areas of his life and previous traumas. He also recognised that learning to forgive his father might take some time, but he was open and keen to work on this using the techniques and tools he learnt during therapy, highlighting how important it is to not only clear traumas, but also integrate the learning, and apply this to his present and future life.*

Summary

- When working spiritually, it is good practice to start observing the energetic connection made with clients from the moment they make contact, during the different areas explored during the history-taking and beyond.
- HLP can be incorporated into the history-taking to provide a BioPsychoSocioSpiritual framework.
- Completing a detailed history with your client enables you to identify their challenges, traumas and attachment/relationship difficulties.
- The next stage is to identify what your client's blocks and restrictions are, as well as the repeated themes throughout their life.
- Identifying positive relationships and resources, which may have a spiritual quality, is also valuable, as these can be installed during the preparation stages.
- Asking your client about their spiritual beliefs as part of your routine history-taking enables you to identify how this can be incorporated into EMDR therapy.

- Discussing the idea of 'energies' is another valuable way of adopting a transpersonal approach, regardless of whether clients are open or not to spirituality.
- Once all relevant information has been obtained, it is important to provide clients with an initial formulation and check to make sure this resonates. This then forms the basis of a treatment plan, which can be re-evaluated throughout EMDR therapy.

Chapter 10

EMDR Phase 2

Preparation A: Resources

'The way is not in the sky; the way is in the heart.'

Buddha

The second phase of EMDR therapy is known as the preparation stage which will be covered over the next two chapters. This chapter focuses on resources and coping strategies that clients can be taught to extend their window of tolerance, including safe/peaceful place, light stream and container exercises along with ideas on how to incorporate these with clients' spiritual beliefs. Additional Resource Development Installation (RDI), which is often needed for the more complex presentations is then discussed, including adding a spiritual quality to the techniques. Resourcing strategies can be introduced during the Phase 1 of EMDR therapy, as well as throughout the EMDR process, to support the stabilisation of clients. Examples of energetic protection and clearing resources, including using different visual exercises, prayers and meditations are then detailed, in order for clients to start taking responsibility for themselves from an energetic and spiritual perspective. Finally, the importance of learning grounding techniques is highlighted.

Resourcing

Safe/calm/peaceful place

Not exclusive to EMDR therapy, the 'safe' place exercise is taught to EMDR therapists during basic training to enable them to teach it to their clients as part of the preparation stage (Shapiro, 2018). It is now widely acknowledged that the word 'safe' can be triggering to some individuals. I use 'peaceful' place, but you could use 'calm place,' 'a place that is special to you' (again, can be triggering for some clients), 'happy' or 'spiritual/sacred place.'

If it is a spiritual or sacred space, then this may be somewhere your client has visited or a location they know about, for example, the Himalayas. It could be in a different healing realm, planet or it may be somewhere visited during meditation and associated with positive feelings that helps them to

DOI: 10.4324/9781003509646-13

self-soothe when they imagine being in this place. They may choose to connect with ascended masters, spirits or deities, energy from nature such as tree spirits, elementals, power animals or multi-dimensional beings such as fairies, dragons, elves and mermaids within this place. For migrants, Spierings (2004) recommend considering using family as the safe place and calling it 'comfortable' rather than safe.

This resource is a very helpful assessment tool because it identifies whether a client is able to self-soothe, connect with and enhance positive feelings in their body. Clients who struggle with this exercise usually need more time during the preparation phase to learn attachment-based resources and mindfulness strategies (especially informal mindfulness), as they tend to be very dissociative and disconnected from physical feelings and emotions. This resource uses mindfulness skills, asking the client to notice what they can see, hear, smell and taste as they deepen their connection to their chosen place. I have worked with a number of clients who may have had EMDR with another clinician and been taught to access a safe/peaceful place, but presented as still very dissociative. Sometimes they had not processed traumas sufficiently in their previous therapy because the dissociation had not been fully addressed. Therefore, I have found that it is beneficial to teach clients informal mindfulness strategies before introducing this exercise so that they understand how to connect with their senses and go deeper into the experience. Otherwise, the safe/peaceful place may at times act as a form of dissociation and avoidance, providing another dissociative technique to take them away from their current reality when they are struggling.

This resource also provides an opportunity to practise BLS (bilateral stimulation), and can be used as part of the client's daily resource toolkit as well as for closing down sessions. Not all clients enjoy or are able to connect with this exercise, so it is important to have a variety of alternative techniques, for example, I have observed clients sometimes preferring the extended light stream exercise (see below).

My current sacred place is an oak tree that I visit on most days and is in the most beautiful location near to where I live, a painting of which is on the front cover of this book. I have had very spiritual experiences in this place, have connected with and seen elementals, and the healing energy in this spot feels extremely powerful to me. I have also heard other people visit this place and call it the sacred tree, so it is interesting that these energies can also be sensed by others.

The New Extended Light Stream

This is probably one of the most favoured resources used by clients, originally described by Shapiro (2001) for stress reduction and chronic pain, whose origins go back to ancient yoga traditions. It is now used with many clients regardless of their presenting problems as part of an ongoing self-care and self-soothing resource. I have adapted and extended the light stream to include:

- Mindful breathing, anchoring the person to the here and now.
- A light stream, where clients are guided to imagine a healing light working its way through the body.
- Grounding techniques, where clients are invited to imagine roots from their feet, like roots from an oak tree, entering the ground and making them feel strong and secure.
- Protection, where clients imagine themselves surrounded by a protective bubble or shield that only allows the entry of positive thoughts and energy.

I have a recording of this on my YouTube channel which anyone can listen to as part of a guided meditation ('The "New" Extended Light Stream' by Alexandra Dent). I have provided the script below in case you would like to record your own version. You can of course change things depending on your client's spiritual beliefs or add words like 'Divine' healing light, God, connecting to Mother Earth or Gaia, sending away anything that is not positive to be transmuted to divine love, etc.

Exercise 7: The New Extended Light Stream meditation exercise

'The first thing I would like you to do is to find a quiet place for the next ten minutes where you will not be disturbed and get into a comfy position, either sitting on a chair or lying down, and if it feels comfortable close your eyes or if you prefer, just settle yourself on a neutral gazing spot in front of you.'

(Pause)

'Then start to bring your attention to your breath and notice the movement of air into and out of your body............. Don't try and speed it up or slow it down............. just accept it is what it is meant to be at this moment in time. Notice the movement of air entering your nose and into your lungs............. and then leaving your lungs............. back through your nose and out of your body. Sometimes it helps to think of the word CALM as you breathe in, ... breathing in the calm into the whole of your body,............. and then think of the words LETTING GO as you breath out, ... breathing out all the stress and tension you may be holding onto inside.'

(Pause)

'Breathing in the calm and then letting go.'

(Pause)

'Now I want you to imagine a beautiful light stream above your head, as if someone is shining down a torch full of the most beautiful healing light. And *ever so gently, I want you to imagine this healing light entering the top of your head and filling your head and face full of this beautiful healing light, filling every cell in your head and face full of this light, very calm and relaxed and letting go of any of the stress and tension, any of the worries that you might be holding on to. Just imagine them all dissolving away and filling that space that is remaining with the healing light.'*

(Pause)

'Once your head and face are full of the light, I want you to imagine that it is gently going to flow down your throat and neck and at your shoulders, I want you to imagine the light separating into two parts; one part flowing down your left arm and the other part flowing down your right arm. Imagine this healing light gently flowing down your arms, relaxing and soothing as it flows, flowing down to your elbows, down to your wrists and hands, and all the way to the tips of your fingers.'

(Pause)

'Then bringing your attention back to your shoulders, I want you to allow more of this healing light to gently flow down the front of your body and down your back, flowing down through your chest and your lungs and your heart, down through your spine and your ribs, gently flowing down through your stomach and your bowels, releasing the tension and stress and just filling that space with this beautiful healing light. Just notice the calmness and relaxation as it flows through your body.'

(Pause)

'At the top of your hips, I want you to again imagine the light separating into two parts; one part going down your left leg, the other part down your right leg. Allow this healing light to gently flow down your legs, down to your knees, down to your ankles and all the way to the tips of your toes, again letting go of any stress or tension you might be holding on to in these areas.'

(Pause)

'Now your whole body is full of this beautiful healing light. Just take a moment or two to notice the wonderful feeling inside your body, like a sunshine glowing, the warmth inside, and just enjoy the feelings it is creating with the healing light flowing around, making sure it reaches every part of your body. Any areas where there might be a slight blockage, just give yourself permission to let go and allow the light to gently dissolve away the stress in that area.'

(Pause)

'Still keeping your eyes closed, I want you to imagine roots coming from the base of your feet, spreading deep, deep down into the earth below, spreading further and further down, making you feel very secure, very strong and

grounded. I want you to imagine your body is like the trunk of a wise old oak tree, full of this healing light, feeling very secure in the ground below.

(Pause)

Now I would like you to imagine that you are surrounded by a protective bubble, a very special bubble that only allows the positive thoughts and moments in life to enter. Any of the negativity or stress from the outside world just bounces off the edge of the bubble, sent back into the universe. The protective bubble surrounds you and allows the good positive, happy thoughts through. You may wish to fill the space between yourself and the edge of your protective bubble with more of the healing light, making you feel even stronger, even more secure.

(Pause)

Holding on to this beautiful image of you being this strong wise oak tree, full of the beautiful healing light shining within, with strong deep roots into the earth and completely surrounded by this very protective bubble, I want you to very gently in your own time, start wiggling your fingers and wiggling your toes, just slowly become aware of the surface that you are lying or sitting on, just start noticing…………. and very gently when you are ready start opening up your eyes and coming back into the room, feeling much more relaxed, calm and very grounded.'

Container exercise

This is another useful resource tool that therapists can use with clients requiring more resourcing strategies and some clients may choose to include a spiritual aspect to this.

Exercise 8: The Container exercise

'I would like you to imagine a container, it could be a cardboard box, trunk, plastic tub, shipping box, wardrobe etc. Try to choose something that is not connected with any previous triggers or traumas. Let me know when you have something to mind and what it is.'

When the client has something in mind and tells you what it is (and you deem it appropriate and not triggering to their situation), then say:

'I would like you to imagine opening your container and putting all the memories and distressing things that have happened to you into your container.'

I ask the client to let me know when this has happened and then get them to double check by scanning their body for any signs of distress or discomfort. If there is anything they detect, then I guide them to put this into the container as well. I then say:

'I would like you to close your container and seal it up however you want, making sure nothing can get out. You may want to wrap it in bubble wrap, cellophane, tape, use bolts, locks or chains.'

Again, I ask the client to let me know when they have managed to do this and then say:

'I would like you to imagine a place that you can take your container, somewhere which isn't triggering for you and that will not impact on you day to day. Sometimes people choose to put it on a rocket and send it into space, drop it into a volcano, bury it on a desert island or drop it into the ocean.'

Ask your client to let you know when they have taken or sent their container somewhere where it can be safely left, then say:

'Now, I would like you to imagine coming away from that place, gently coming further and further away until you can no longer sense, see or feel your container.'

After the client has managed to let the connection with their container go, I ask them what that feels like inside their body. Hopefully, they will have a positive feeling or emotion and I ask them to notice where they feel this in their body and then use a set of slow, short BLS as they connect with the positive felt sense. I continue this for a few sets if they report positive feedback. I then ask them to think of a word or phrase that goes along with that feeling and install this using another set of slow, short BLS (similar to the safe/peaceful place exercise). This is another helpful exercise to use with some clients to see how able they are to disconnect from some of the distress they are experiencing, even for a short time, and whether they can connect with more positive feelings in their body. If not, then further resource and attachment work is required before moving on to EMDR processing.

For spiritually minded clients, the container itself may be of spiritual significance, for example, a healing box, old sacred container (maybe a vase or chalice), or the client may choose to put crystals, aromatherapy oils or a healing scent such as sage, inside the container. It could be sealed and protected with prayers, healing spells, mantras or spiritual deities who are recognised for their protective qualities, like Archangel Michael. The container could be taken to a spiritual realm, temple, place in nature or planet that is of significance and meaning to the client, or put in the care of the Divine, God, Buddha, Allah, and so forth. Adapt as resonates with your client and you could make some suggestions for them if they needed support or guidance. One client of mine used a container with some healing crystals inside and a Reiki symbol on the outside to act as protection. She then imagined sending this container, with all her distressing memories to a nearby nature reserve and buried it underneath an oak tree.

Be creative with this exercise and adapt it for different cultures so that it resonates with the client's own belief systems. Adaptations may include using baskets, pots, bags, instead of the word 'container '(Mbazzi et al., 2021). You could use a literal box when doing the container exercise for example, a mesob (food container), or a jerry can (something that is familiar to them that is hardwearing and strong). Clients may choose to have the container within the clinic setting, or it may be an actual physical container which they can put stones, pebbles or another suitable object in to help them leave this behind after a session. Perhaps your client could bury a meaningful object or symbol in some sand (if this is available in your setting), use a healing crystal alongside the container or object, say a prayer, mantra, smudge with sage to clear negative energies, or perform another meaningful protective ritual. Some clients, including children, may find it helpful to draw something and leave this in a book or envelope with the therapist who can take care of it until the next appointment. Of course, it's important for you to make an accurate record of what the client has chosen so that you and they can reconnect with it in future sessions if required.

Resource Development Installation

Leeds (1998) and Korn & Leeds (2002) introduced the term Resource Development Installation (RDI) to describe the technique of helping clients with complex issues to regulate their affect, which may include mastery, relational or symbolic resources. Mastery resources represent times in a person's life where clients were successful, achieved something, set appropriate, healthy boundaries, managed to engage with positive self-care or were able to be assertive or speak their truth. Relational resources help the client to connect with times when they were able to successfully access support in their life (care, guidance, empathy, etc.), or had helpful role models, demonstrating capabilities or positive ways of being that the client would like to embrace. Role models do not necessarily need to be someone the client has known and can include historic or fictional figures, but the qualities held by that role model must have significance and positive meaning for them. Symbolic resources can come from a variety of cultural, spiritual or metaphysical sources including dreams, art, music, and so forth.

Examples of RDI may include connecting to a time when your client felt a positive sense during a spiritual experience, either during a healing session, on a spiritual retreat, in nature, listening to mantras, mudras, in pray or meditation.

In her book *Tapping in*, Parnell (2008) provided many ways of installing resources to help manage difficult emotions and traumas. She advocated that we are essentially whole and have everything we need within us (something I also believe) and that we can learn to connect to the inner, positive, healing resources within to activate and strengthen this, including accessing nurturing, protective and wise figures, which can be particularly helpful for clients who have experienced early attachment difficulties. Such groups of figures can include individuals who are known to a person, animals, spiritual figures or someone they know about from a book, film or who are historical figures. Clients are encouraged to connect within and bring up the qualities (either nurturing, protective or wise) as they think of a particular figure, including using their senses to notice what they see, hear, feel and smell. Once this is established and a strong sense is achieved, this can be 'tapped in' using a slow set of BLS, continuing for a few sets if the feelings get stronger. A circle of protective figures can also be installed by imagining all the protective figures that have already been tapped in surrounding the client, and then install this with BLS. I sometimes invite a person to imagine their heart and soul connecting with the heart and soul of the respective figures in their protective circle and tap this in too. Parnell also provides scripts for resourcing angels who represent nurturing figures, as well as inner wisdom figures, various meditations, tapping in spiritually positive experiences, connections with higher self or a higher source.

Some of the spiritual resources I regularly use include imagining myself being surrounded, protected and embraced by Archangel Michael's wings or being in the warmth, protection and energy of the Divine. I also find comfort when connecting with an image of Jesus carrying the cross, as this illustrates to me that even in great hardship or distress, Jesus found the strength to keep going. In addition, I connect with Mother Mary and her nurturing and unconditional love, which provides me with a sense of comfort, support and strength.

Protecting and clearing energies

This is something that I often use with clients where they are either struggling to have healthy boundaries with their energy, feel others are siphoning their energy, or they feel they are absorbing projections from those around them. I love the Harry Potter stories by J.K. Rowling and I personally think there are so many wonderful ideas that can be adapted from these books for protecting energies.

Protective bubble/cloak

In this exercise, clients are invited to imagine being surrounded by a protective cloak or protective bubble that only allows the positive healing energies to enter. Anything that is not in alignment with high vibrational positive emotions from their environment, or from others, is rebounded from the edge of the cloak or bubble so that it cannot enter the energy space. I have included this as part of the New Extended Light Stream exercise as described earlier.

Another technique I have found personally helpful, is that when I become aware that someone is sending negative energy to me, I metaphorically imagine my hand extending in front of me to the place where the energy feels like it is being directed at me to act as a barrier, and an internal voice inside me says 'No.' In this way, I am consciously confronting the energy head on and refusing to absorb it into my energy field.

Patronus spell

Informed from J.K. Rowling's Harry Potter books, this resource can be adapted as required. The idea is that if one feels like they are being sent projected negative energies, they can imagine a healing light energy or variant of a Patronus (a character, symbol or animal, etc. of their choosing that has a positive protective quality to it), to deter and repel the projections and negative energy away.

Mirrors

Ask the client to imagine they are surrounded by mirrors facing outwards and that anything being sent to them by another person, that does not originate from high emotional vibrations such as joy, bliss, love and light, is reflected back to the sender. If possible, invite your client to reflect this energy back with love. We do not want to encourage our clients to connect with anger, hurt or pain, otherwise they can get caught in a destructive energy battle with the other person. Alternatively, if your client is concerned about reflecting back the projections to the original sender, you could ask them to divert any projected energy in to the universe or Divine, asking that the energy is transmuted into healing light and love.

Heart connection and meditation

Another technique that I have found particularly useful and also teach to clients is using a heart meditation, whether it is one of the guided short Heartmath meditations on my YouTube channel ('Quick Coherence Technique ^{TM}' by Alexandra Dent, or 'Heart Focused Breathing^{TM}' by Alexandra Dent) or one that you create yourself.

If I notice negative energies in my environment, and feel this is starting to impact on my own energies, I try to find a moment to remove myself and seek out a quiet, calm space. I tune into my energies and notice whether I may have absorbed some of this negative energy. Have I started feeling angry, stressed or sad whereas before I was feeling okay? I then connect in my heart and use my breath to breathe into and out of my heart area to release and transmute any lower vibrational emotions. Next, I intentionally connect with higher vibrational energies of love, joy, bliss and grace, breathing those into and out of my heart area. Finally, I bring the person or situation to mind that was holding the distress, and send love from my heart. I have found that it is best to go through these stages rather than to bypass any stage, as it is important to facilitate transmutation of the distress first. In this way, when I imagine connecting with the person or situation, it is with pure unconditional love. Personally, I have noticed and been amazed by how much quicker relationships can be resolved or healed when I have tried this exercise, especially with my children!

Hawaiian Ho'oponopono forgiveness prayer

This is a lovely Hawaiian prayer for forgiveness which is beautiful and incredibly powerful. Remember that our thoughts and intentions create energy. Connecting with the words in this short prayer and sending them to a person you may be having conflict or challenges with can be transformative. I try to hold the intention of coming from a place of healing to clear the energy and improve the relationship and dynamics. I use this regardless of whether I could interpret or perceive the situation as me being the victim or not; I try not to engage with that energy as that is ego-based. The word *ho'oponopono* roughly translates to 'cause things to move back in to balance' or 'to make things right.'

'I am sorry.
Please forgive me.
Thank you.
I love you.'

Protection and clearing prayer

This is a short prayer that you can use either for yourself as part of your daily self-care as well as give to your clients. The aim is to facilitate clearing any energies or projections that may have attached to your energy field. My rule of thumb is that if I notice a change in my mood or beliefs, I reflect on whether this is triggering my inner wounds or parts, whether I may be picking up energies from the collective, or whether I have been in contact with someone and absorbed their energies or projections. This means I am attempting to adopt a constant state of self-enquiry throughout the day. If it is my material, I mindfully go within and befriend what has come up, use various techniques to allow the energy to flow through me, and remain open to learning and integrating important lessons of what the experience is showing me. If it feels more like collective energies, then I still connect with it but I am less attached to the details of what it is and allow it to flow through me. If I feel that I may have absorbed projections, then I will use the following clearing prayer to help release these from my energy field.

'Angels, teachers and guides. Please open a portal above my head to the Divine now. Angels, teachers and guides, please remove any energies that are not mine and send them through the portal now. Please transmute all that energy into divine love.'

Allow sufficient time for the clearing to happen. During this, you might notice a release of energy, some movement in your energy field, or you might notice nothing, and that is okay too. Just give it a little time, observe and allow whatever needs to happen to happen. It is really important to finish by closing down the portal, otherwise you are keeping your energy field open. The portal is closed by saying:

'Thank you, angels, teachers and guides. Please close the portal now.'

Please amend the wording so that it resonates with your client's belief system (or yours if you are using this for yourself). For example, you could open a portal to God, other deities, other healing dimensions etc. You could invite ancestors or other parts of one's support team to assist with this clearing too. Alternatively, if your client likes praying, they could pray to their chosen healing source and asked for any negative energies that do not belong to them or are not in their highest good to be cleared from their body.

With all of the exercises mentioned in this chapter, if the situation doesn't change, ask your client to reflect on the relationships they have that are still causing them distress. Using the resources above is not about enabling toxic relationships to continue by the client acting as the rescuer of constantly trying to heal others. When these situations arise repeatedly, it is worth asking your client to reflect on what is being shown to them. Are their people or situations no longer aligned with them at this stage in their journey? Is the vibrational energy of some others no longer compatible with theirs, without trying to specify whether theirs is higher or lower, because again that may be coming from a place of ego? Do they feel drained or distressed much of the time in someone's presence? If so, then the energy, whether it is emotional, cognitive, physical or spiritual is trying to communicate something to them. Do they need to reconsider the role this person is having in their life, and does that need changing or ending? If a change is required, are they struggling to have confidence or self-worth to make the change, or is there a deeper soul level block that is preventing them for making the necessary changes? If this is the case, then it is highly likely the dynamics will continue, regardless of what energetic or protective resources they put in place.

All of these protective and clearing resources can be performed anywhere and at any time quietly in one's own mind, without having to be explicit or obvious about what is being done. I encourage clients to become mindful of their energies as well as practice various self-care and protection techniques as they navigate difficult circumstances. Sometimes this includes teaching them the protective prayer very early on in sessions, perhaps during the first or second appointment, even if I have not completed the initial assessment. This usually happens when the clients are either still attempting to leave, or have recently left, toxic relationships (possibly due to family circumstances or finances), and their energy fields are very open, thus soaking up the projections and negative energy from others. Often, when I am teaching the client the protective prayer, Light Language comes through to facilitate the transmutation of some of the negative energies. An example of this is with one client who was working through a very acrimonious divorce said: 'Amazing, that is so powerful, I now feel I can handle the situation.' At the following session, she reported how the conversation around energy and protection had helped her greatly in making important decisions, including installing healthier, energetic boundaries in her life.

Case example: Lilly and energy protection resources

Lilly was introduced previously in Chapter 2. *She had really started to inte-grate her self-care strategies, including protective energy techniques, noticing an improvement in overall anxiety levels, as well as her ability to manage ongoing challenging situations. The EMDR processing was helping reduce anxiety from the numerous hospital procedures and chronic physical health issues experienced she was a child, as well as targeting complex relationships with family members. Throughout her life, Lilly had often been used as the middle person in her parents' complex relationship. Her father had underlying mental health issues and she also worked in the family business. We had dowsed Lilly's life lesson which was 'healing' and we explored how this could be experienced in many different ways; learning to trust that she had healing abilities that she could practise on herself and possibly for others in the future, learning when to receive healing from others (including therapy) and when to step away from being in the healing role (not soaking up others projections) when this was to her own detriment.*

Lilly arrived at one session feeling more overwhelmed than usual. She dis-cussed how her father had been for a hospital procedure the week before and how her mother had been in a terribly anxious state. All of this was impacting on Lilly significantly and we were able to identify how her mother was pro-jecting distress into Lilly, a regular occurrence, including belittling her in front of colleagues at work. Lilly had once again found herself caught up in her parents' distress and had forgotten to use some of her protection and resource techniques. She was able to recognise that she was internalising the barrage of abuse from her mother, which subsequently was making her feel overwhelmed, and she could identify how she was acting yet again as the sponge for her par-ents' issues. In our session, Lilly was able to reflect on how her mother reg-ularly accused her own mother (maternal grandmother) of similar behaviours, but was completely unaware or unable to take any ownership for what she was projecting on to Lilly. I supported Lilly to step outside this recent drama and observe herself energetically, noticing what this situation was trying to show or teach her from an HLP perspective. Lilly reflected on how it was a repeated lesson for her to be more empowered and protect her own energies, rather than healing other people's distress at her own expense. We proceeded with the protection prayer to clear her energetic space and were then in a position to target an upcoming significant hospital procedure using EMDR, connecting with her universal support team before we started.

Grounding

Learning grounding techniques, including mindfulness (informal techniques) and mindful breathing, is an essential part of the spiritual journey as part of ongoing self-care, and is also beneficial when preparing clients for EMDR, especially those who dissociate. Other grounding techniques include using crystals, aromatherapy oils, scents, connecting with the earth, for example, walking bare foot on grass or soil, gardening and walking in nature. In some cultures, using drumming, clapping, rhythm and movement, dance, song and toe-tapping can be very grounding, especially if these are in alignment with an individual's belief system. Apparently, having a piece of chocolate (especially dark chocolate) can be grounding as well as other food types including root vegetables and red foods. It is always a good idea to have a glass of water available for clients, as this can be a quick way to help ground them – and yourself – during the session.

The energy that a client brings into the room can have an impact on how the session progresses, and whilst you may be doing your best to provide a safe, containing environment, if they arrive scattered or ungrounded, then it is likely to impact on the spiritual resonance and energy in the session. I tend to gently name what is happening so that the client can learn more awareness about the shifts and changes in energy and learn how to modify these to be in their window of tolerance and get the most out of a session. An example of this is when Mary arrived at her second session in an elevated mood, saying she was feeling 'very excitable.' Mary described herself as a spiritually attuned and insightful lady, embracing her journey and making changes from ego to heart led living in order to 'walk the walk' and be more aligned with her authenticity. I suggested practising some grounding techniques to help calm her energies to which she was in agreement. Mary started connecting to her breath and gave me permission to use the root chakra crystal sound bowl. She reported absorbing the energetic vibrations from the sound bowl and I sensed her energies were calming. I felt Light Language coming through, and with her agreement, I channelled a few minutes and noticed us both aligning more in the energetic space. I had never spoken Light Language to her before and asked her how she felt after this and the crystal bowl. She looked quite emotional, hands on her heart and said she felt 'pure love, more centred, calm and grounded.' At the end of the session, Mary commented on how grounded she was still feeling.

Summary

- Teaching clients resources not only prepares them for EMDR desensitisation, but also introduces them to essential coping skills that they can continue to utilise whilst navigating their spiritual journey.
- Spiritual ideas can be incorporated into the different traditional resource exercises to align with your clients' beliefs. This can prove to be a very powerful ongoing support for them.
- Different protection and clearing techniques, including using different visual exercises, prayers and meditations, can assist clients to start taking

greater responsibility for their own energies both from within themselves and as part of their extended energetic field.

- As clients learn to care for themselves energetically, they will also adopt healthier boundaries in relationships and situations which may otherwise have drained them.
- It is important that clients learn how to ground their energies as this keeps them more connected to the present moment.

Chapter 11

EMDR Phase 2

Preparation B: Part work, soul level work, rebirthing procedure and narrative EMDR

'Out of difficulties grow miracles.'

Jean de la Bruyère

This chapter continues with resources that may be required for more complex clients during the preparation stage of EMDR with particular focus on soul level work. An overview of traditional part work therapy is first discussed. How to work at a soul level is then covered, including four initial steps to consider at the beginning of these sessions. This is followed by two detailed scripts on how to support clients to either connect with their spiritual home in order to obtain guidance with their current incarnation, or to reclaim lost soul parts or fragments. A rebirthing procedure is provided for those clients who have experienced in utero or birth trauma and this is illustrated with a case example. All of the techniques described have emerged based on my own personal healing and clinical practice over many years. Finally, the value of incorporating a spiritual approach when using EMDR attachment narratives is discussed and scripts are provided that can be used for adolescents, adults and refugees. Some adaptations for the younger person are also mentioned.

Part work and inner child work

This is a fantastic way of working with dissociative clients to prepare them for EMDR processing and is often an essential pre-requisite for the more complex cases. We all have parts to us, whether they represent the lighter aspects of ourselves such as fun, loving, nurturing, supportive, friendly parts or aspects of our shadow side including suicidal, sabotage, angry, hurtful, lonely, shame, despair, distrust and neglectful parts, etc. The challenge arises when different parts are in conflict with each other, have dissociative barriers in place and are not working together as a supportive team. Learning over time to have compassion, love and to welcome and embrace all parts of ourselves is a key part of the spiritual journey; the light and shadow sides. From a spiritual perspective, part work may involve healing difficulties from the present lifetime as well as past lives, ancestral wounds, understanding archetypes

DOI: 10.4324/9781003509646-14

or soul level retrieval. There is no quick fix or spiritual bypassing for this stage as that simply creates a lack of authenticity in one's life. It is not an easy process and therefore takes considerable time.

There are many highly effective therapies that focus on part work including Internal Family Systems, Ego State work, Schema Therapy and Gestalt Therapy. I believe it comes down to personal choice and finding your own truth as to what resonates to you and your client rather than saying one approach is better than the other. You may be trained in several of these therapies, adapting and utilising them according to your client's presentation.

I have undergone training in various Ego State courses since 2013 as this approach really resonated with me and has helped develop my confidence and skillset in working with dissociative clients. It provided a safe, containing technique to support clients to meet their different parts so that they could learn to form healthier relationships between those different parts. It also marked the beginning of my interest and development in inner child work (younger self work) as often a person's inner child/children would emerge during these sessions. It provided an opportunity to build the relationship between the client and their inner child parts, especially at a heart and soul level. I invited clients to recognise and learn to connect with the infinite bond between their heart and their inner child's heart and encourage clients to practise this on a daily basis. Areas of HLP, such as learning self-compassion, self-worth, self-love and authenticity, were deepened as the client formed a more positive and healing relationship with their inner child. I encouraged clients to teach their inner child, or different parts of themselves, various resources including spiritual energy protection, clearing and healing work as they journeyed along their spiritual path together. I also learnt to bring in spiritual qualities to these sessions when client's parts were ready to integrate, allowing their different energy fields and auras to merge.

It was several years later when I was undergoing a great deal of my own soul level healing with both Akashic Records, shamanic healing and soul retrieval that I realised that there was a parallel between the techniques used for these spiritual therapies and the Ego State work I was using. I remember reflecting back to my shamanic practitioner that I felt we were doing similar processes in our work; hers in a more 'alternative therapy' practice and mine in a more traditional psychotherapy practice. She would use the word 'soul fragment' instead of 'part work' to describe similar methods. We both used a visual meditation to guide a person into a safe place, usually a house that metaphorically represented themselves, before meeting the different parts. On reflection, what was different was that my shamanic practitioner was intentionally working at a soul level whereas I had not integrated this into my clinical work at the time. Therefore, if appropriate and with their agreement, this opened up a deeper way of supporting clients to work at a soul level and reclaim soul fragments that had broken off as a consequence of various traumas, whether in this life or in past lives.

During Ego State sessions, I have assisted some clients to float back to past lives to identify soul level blocks that may still be impacting on their current life. This provided a chance to learn what the life lesson was and make new choices to move forwards in their journey. It also helped identify past life work that may be a target for future EMDR processing.

Working at a soul level

There are many different, creative ways that we can intentionally work at a soul level with our clients and here I am going to discuss just a few. I acknowledge there are EMDR therapists who already work in this way and may have developed their own style and ideas. I am sure as time progresses and therapists become more comfortable in working spiritually, these ideas will continue to expand and adapt. The information, different scripts and techniques provided below are suggestions to support those therapists who prefer some structure.

This work is applicable for those clients who resonate with a soul or essence and I do not suggest embarking on this if the client does not believe in these concepts as it will feel invasive and likely rupture the therapeutic relationship. Some clients who are embracing a spiritual journey may not need to have different spiritual procedures as the standard (or modified) EMDR protocol will allow them to access the places and knowledge spontaneously. They will naturally be able to connect with spirits, past lives, ascended masters or other deities (see Daniel's case study in Chapter 13).

Therapist being in alignment with their soul

When working at a soul level, it is important that the therapist embraces being in alignment with their soul as they undertake their spiritual journey. How can you expect your clients to complete soul level work with you if you are not striving towards a healthy, healing relationship with your own soul? The client's soul will not feel safe, contained or have trust in you. You must act as a role model for your clients. I also believe that working at a soul level means tapping into a different energetic healing space, frequency and vibration, enabling the possibility of multi-dimensional healing. Therefore, ensuring there is some protection around both you and your client and setting the intentions of the space that you will be connecting with is crucial. Ideas on how to do this have already been discussed in Chapters 2 and 10.

If you are planning on carrying out past life or soul level work regularly with clients, I would strongly recommend that you undergo additional soul level training and your own personal healing in these areas so that you have a greater understanding of the process and can support your client effectively. This may include undertaking Akashic Record healing, Past Life Regression, Shamanic training, soul level retrieval, Beyond Quantum Healing or other similar modalities. Of course, I also appreciate that clients may naturally connect to past lives without it having been an explicit intent of the session. If this happens, the client is most likely feeling energetically safe enough with you to do this, so trust the process and don't panic. Clients may only need to dip in to the past life briefly just to make an adaptive connection before naturally returning to this lifetime. If in doubt, or you are not feeling competent, then gently guide the client to connect back to the original memory in this current lifetime that you started with. It is not advisable to begin a conversation about what they are experiencing if they do slip into past lives as this will break the flow of the processing. Your job is to be their navigator and to keep out of the way as much as possible, irrespective of the curiosity of your own ego. Remember that whilst there may be a level of curiosity from both parts, it is not usually helpful to try and over-analyse what happens at the end of the session as this can make the client become attached to the experience rather than just allow its release. The key focus is to establish the meaning for the client that can enable them to integrate the learning.

Soul level work

If you and your client have agreed to complete some soul level EMDR processing then it is important to make sure you have agreement with their soul that they are willing to engage in this healing; making it explicit brings it into the client's conscious awareness. They are not just having something 'done' to them, they are an active participant.

It is important to have some idea about the client's intentions before completing soul level work. Questions they would like to explore and obtain guidance with may include:

- What is their soul purpose?
- Information about life lessons.
- Spiritual support team and resources available to them in this lifetime.
- Understanding about certain challenges or relationships that they have experienced.
- Possible past life traumas and the impact these may still be having on current incarnation.

These are the four initial steps that I would recommend considering at the beginning of sessions before proceeding with soul level work.

1   Ask for agreement from the client and their soul/essence to work on the presenting trauma.
2   Create a protective energetic space for you and your client. This may be something pertinent to them or connecting with the Divine Source and asking for a protective barrier to surround you and your client. You may choose to use one of the protection examples provided in Chapters 2 and 10.

3   Check that all parts of the client are happy to work on the trauma. If not, then invite those parts that are unwilling to participate and to retreat to their safe/peaceful/calm/sacred place where they can rest until the session has been completed.

4   Here are some additional stages which you can encourage your client to do:

-   Connect with the quantum field where all possibilities exist.
-   Connect with their spiritual resource team which may include spiritual, nurturing, protective and wise figures, power animals, their Akashic Records, etc.
-   Connect with their breath and intentionally breathe into the heart and/or soul area. You could use one of the scripts provided in Chapters 5 and 6.
-   Imagine a healing cord or line flowing from their heart, downwards through their body into Mother Earth, to feel grounded.
-   Imagine a healing cord or line going from their heart, upwards through the top of their body, and connecting with a place of their choice (Divine, God, Buddha, Allah, Sun, Moon, particular healing realm, etc.).
-   If you are trained in Akashic Record healing, then with your client's permission you could connect with their Akashic Records. Remember to close down the Akashic Records once the work is complete.

Below are scripts for two different options of soul level work; connecting to client's spiritual home and reclaiming soul fragments/parts. They are adapted from the Ego State training I attended, as well as my own personal experience of having soul retrieval sessions. I would be cautious about using this for the younger teenagers and definitely do not recommend this for young children. Please adapt according to your client's culture or belief system.

Connecting to clients' spiritual home

I have tried this process when a client has been struggling to integrate other forms of soul healing and therapies and there is a sense that their soul is not really wanting to be embodied within the human experience in this incarnation. You would use it in the preparation phase if you intuitively sense that the client is unlikely to be able to process trauma until they have a greater awareness of their spiritual journey or feel their soul may dissociate because they are struggling to be embodied in physical form in this lifetime. However, this may not become obvious until the assessment or desensitisation phases, and if this is the case, I would pause further processing and consider completing the soul level work first. This technique can also help if your client would like to gain more information about their soul's choices before incarnation or connect with their soul spiritual support team. They may seek guidance as to the reasons why they chose to incarnate in this current lifetime, the traumas, challenges and relationships they have experienced, their various life lessons as well as their soul purpose.

If the client has NCs such as:

- I don't trust my soul, or,
- I didn't choose to incarnate, or,
- My spiritual journey is too much, I can't succeed,

then this may indicate that they would benefit from connecting back to their spiritual home and gaining some insight and wisdom that can facilitate them in their spiritual journey.

Instructions for connecting to clients' spiritual home

'I would like you to get yourself into a really nice comfortable position sitting down, legs uncrossed, feet on the floor, rest your hands on your lap and if it feels comfortable close your eyes, or if you prefer, just settle yourself on a neutral gazing spot in front of you.'

(Pause)

'Start to bring your awareness to the movement of the breath into and out of your body............ notice how the air enters your nose into your lungs............. and then back out from your lungs through your nose into the room again............. Don't try to speed it up or slow it down, just allow it to be whatever it needs to be in this moment in time.'

(Pause)

'Allow the breath to anchor you in this moment.'

(Pause)

'I would like you to imagine that you are standing by a gate that opens up into a beautiful garden and there is a house in the garden that feels very familiar and safe to you. This is a space that is just for you and feels very calm and peaceful. When you are ready, I would like you to open the gate and step into the garden, closing the gate behind you. Take a look around and notice what you can see, smell, hear, feel as you stand in your garden. Notice if there are clouds in the sky, if the sun is shining, if it is a warm or cool day, if there is a gentle breeze or whether the air feels still. Notice if you can hear any birds or insects, what kind of plants or shrubs are in your garden. Just notice.'

(Pause)

'Become aware of a garden path that runs from the gate you have entered to the front door of the house and I would like you to start walking along this path to the

house. Notice what type of house it is, whether it is made of bricks, stones, wood or something else. Notice how many windows you can see, whether there are chimney pots and any other features of the house. As you arrive at the front door, again notice what type of door it is, what type of door handle it has. Take a few breaths just to feel very grounded and connected to this space.'

(Pause)

'When you are ready, I would like you to open the door and step inside the house and close the door behind you. Notice the airy hallway, whether it has a tiled or wooden floor, slabs or something else, maybe some rugs. There may be a staircase leading upstairs. Notice if the hallway has any mirrors, paintings or plants within.'

(Pause)

'From the hallway there are several doors that lead to different rooms and you are instinctively drawn to one. Open the door and step inside into a large, light, calm, safe room, closing the door behind you. In the middle of this room are some comfy chairs and sofas. Take a moment to acquaint yourself with the furniture and objects in the room. Notice how many windows there are, if there is a fireplace, plants or mirrors. When you are ready, walk towards the centre of the room and take a seat in one of the comfy chairs and take a few slow deep breaths to ground yourself in this moment.'

(Pause)

'This room is a very safe and secure place that you can connect to your soul and spiritual support team. When you are ready, bring your awareness into your heart and/or soul and connect with any of your support team that you would like assistance from today that can provide some guidance for you on your current life spiritual journey. This may include connecting to ascended masters, the Divine, God, guides, Archangels, Gods or Goddesses, dragons, fairies, elementals etc that resonate with you (amend according to the client's cultural and belief system). *Let me know when you have a connection.'*

If the client is struggling to connect you could use the following instructions:

'There are a number of other doors leading in to the room which you are currently seated. I would like you to send out the intention to meet your soul or spiritual support team and as you do this you may notice one or several of the doors open. Who or what do you notice entering the room?'

Allow time for the client to give you feedback about who or what has come forwards to assist in this session. When the client has a connection, I would ask permission to introduce myself, saying:

'My name is {insert your name} and I am supporting {insert client's name} to help them understand and process some of the challenges and difficulties they have been experiencing. Thank you so much for coming today to support them in

this process. If there is anything you are unsure about or would like to ask, then please feel free to let {insert client's name} or me know.'

Invite the client to connect with their support team and they may instinctively ask questions that are relevant to their chosen intention for the session. If, however, they need some guidance, then possible questions you can suggest they may wish to ask their soul or spiritual support team include:

- 'What is the main life lesson I chose to experience this lifetime and why?'
- 'What are the reasons why I chose to experience (name a specific trauma or traumas)?'
- 'What are the reasons why (name a specific person or relationship) is in my life? Is there a joint lesson between them and myself and what is it? Are we both here as teachers for each other or one is more the learner or healer in this relationship?'
- 'What is my soul purpose or mission?'
- 'What spiritual support is available in this lifetime that I am not accessing at the moment?'
- 'What can I start embracing in my life to facilitate my spiritual journey that I may not already be doing?'
- 'How did I feel about incarnating in this lifetime?'
- 'Is there a past life trauma or soul level block that needs releasing to facilitate progress on this incarnation and if so, what is it (this could be a target for future processing)?'

If incarnating into this lifetime did not feel a very positive decision, then you could invite them to converse with their soul or spiritual support team to understand the reasons why it was felt important to incarnate and what support is available to them that they may not be accessing already.

If there is any distress such as anger, sadness, loneliness or despair, and you have previously used BLS with your client, you could consider using BLS to process this negative affect. The client may also connect with a distressing memory or moment, such as when their soul left their spiritual home to incarnate into this lifetime, which could be a target for EMDR processing during a future session. If it feels appropriate and you have time, then you could always process this now.

Once your client has obtained as much information or answers to their questions as possible then it is important to close down the session in a safe and contained manner.

To close the guided exercise, say to the client:

'I would like to thank your spiritual support team for coming today and offering guidance. Remember that you have an infinite, unbreakable cord between you, your soul and your soul's support team that continues beyond the session.'

If the client's soul or spiritual support team had entered through a door, then invite them to leave via that door. Then say to the client:

'I invite you to start bringing your awareness to the movement of the breath into and out of your body.'

(Pause)

'When you are ready, stand up and move towards the door that you initially entered, opening it up and stepping into the light, airy hallway. Then start to walk towards the front door of your house and open it up, stepping out into your garden and closing the front door behind. Take a few slow breaths of fresh air and connect with your senses as you notice your surroundings in the garden.'

(Pause)

'Now start to walk down the pathway that leads from your house to the garden gate, taking in the surrounding scenery. When you arrive at the gate, open it up and step through, closing the gate behind you.'

(Pause)

'I would like you to start wiggling your fingers and toes, notice the surface of what you are sitting on and gently start opening up your eyes into the room you are in and back in to the session with me today.'

Make sure you leave enough time for a debrief and ensure your client in grounded, using any of the resources that you have previously taught them. You could also identify a positive statement by asking them what the most important positive or meaningful part that they can take away from this exercise and install with a few, short slow sets of BLS. Examples include:

- I am learning to understand my soul purpose.
- I am learning to understand or I am open to my spiritual journey.
- I am learning to understand my life lesson.
- I am learning to trust my soul.
- I am learning to embrace this incarnation.
- I am learning to accept myself and the soul level choices I made.
- I have all the resources and support I need.

Reclaiming lost soul parts or fragments

Shamans recognise that clients may still be impacted by parts of a soul that may have fragmented away during severe trauma in past or current lifetimes. Again, I must emphasise that if you are planning on doing this work, make sure you are working within your capabilities and knowledge set and have some training or experience in soul level healing.

Follow the initial four steps in the soul level section described earlier. It is important that the client is consciously aware of the intentions of this exercise which is to reconnect with lost or fragmented parts of their soul.

Instructions for reclaiming lost parts or fragments of the soul

'I would like you to get yourself into a really nice comfortable position sitting down, legs uncrossed, feet on the floor, rest your hands on your lap and if it feels comfortable close your eyes, or if you prefer, just settle yourself on a neutral gazing spot in front of you.'

(Pause)

'Start to bring your awareness to the movement of the breath into and out of your body............ notice how the air enters your nose into your lungs............ and then back out from your lungs through your nose into the room again............. Don't try to speed it up or slow it down, just allow it to be whatever it needs to be in this moment in time.'

(Pause)

'Allow the breath to anchor you in this moment.'

(Pause)

'I would like you to imagine that you are standing by a gate that opens up into a beautiful garden and there is a house in the garden that feels very familiar and safe to you. This is a space that is just for you and feels very calm and peaceful. When you are ready, I would like you to open the gate and step into the garden, closing the gate behind you. Take a look around and notice what you can see, smell, hear, feel as you stand in your garden. Notice if there are clouds in the sky, if the sun is shining, if it is a warm or cool day, if there is a gentle breeze or whether the air feels still. Notice if you can hear any birds or insects, what kind of plants or shrubs are in your garden. Just notice.'

(Pause)

'Become aware of a garden path that runs from the gate you have entered to the front door of the house and I would like you to start walking along this path to the house. Notice what type of house it is, whether it is made of bricks, stones, wood or something else. Notice how many windows you can see, whether there are chimney pots and any other features of the house. As you arrive at the front door, again notice what type of door it is, what type of door handle it has. Take a few breaths just to feel very grounded and connected to this space.'

(Pause)

'When you are ready, I would like you to open the door and step inside the house and close the door behind you. Notice the airy hallway, whether it has a

tiled or wooden floor, slabs or something else, maybe some rugs. There may be a staircase leading upstairs. Notice if the hallway has any mirrors, paintings or plants within.'

(Pause)

'From the hallway there are several doors that lead to different rooms and you are instinctively drawn to one. Open the door and step inside into a large, light, calm, safe room, closing the door behind you. In the middle of this room are some comfy chairs and sofas. Take a moment to acquaint yourself with the furniture and objects in the room. Notice how many windows there are, if there is a fireplace, plants or mirrors. When you are ready walk towards the centre of the room and take a seat in one of the comfy chairs and take a few slow deep breaths to ground yourself in this moment.'

(Pause)

'This room is a very safe and secure place where you can identify whether there are any lost or fragmented parts of your soul, either from previous lifetimes or from this lifetime. There are a number of other doors leading into the room where you are currently seated. When you are ready, bring your awareness into your heart and soul and send out the intention for any lost soul parts that are ready to come forth and join you in the room. What do you notice?'

(Pause)

Allow time for the client to give you feedback about what they notice. It may be that a part (child or adult) appears from a past life or current life, or they sense an energy, shape or just a feeling or presence. When the client has a connection, I would ask permission to introduce myself, saying:

'My name is {insert your name} and I am supporting {insert clients name} to help them understand and process some of the challenges and difficulties they have been experiencing during this incarnation. Thank you so much for coming today to support them in this process. If there is anything you are unsure about or would like to ask, then please feel free to let {insert clients name} or me know. If there is a name you would like to be known as then please let me know.'

This is an opportunity for the client to ask or explore various questions with the soul part to understand what happened that caused the separation or fragmentation. Try to create a compassionate and supportive environment between the client and the soul part. The soul part may be feeling very anxious, afraid, lonely, sad or angry about what happened to them and this is an opportunity to hear how courageous they have been to come forth into the session. If you are familiar with a particular part work therapy then you can use the various techniques that can help build up the relationships and ener-getic connection between the client and the soul parts such as the loving eyes technique (Knipe, 2015). You can bring in HLP concepts for the client to explore with the soul fragments/parts. Questions you can invite your client to explore include:

- 'Did the trauma that resulted in some soul fragmentation happen in this incarnation or another incarnation?'
- 'What happened that caused part of the soul to break away during the trauma?'
- 'Are there any details about this trauma or incarnation that would be helpful to know to help heal the trauma?'
- 'What was the life lesson that you were working on during this challenge and what was this life lesson trying to teach you from a heart perspective?'
- 'What is the gift that can be attained and integrated from this trauma?'
- 'How can you apply this gained knowledge and wisdom moving forwards in this current lifetime when you encounter new challenges?'
- 'What support or resources does the soul fragment/part need to help them feel ready to re-integrate?'

How much work required for the soul fragment/part to be heard, understood and ready to integrate back in to the client may depend on the complexity of the trauma experienced by the soul fragment/part and this may take several sessions. Try not to have any expectations or rush the process, and offer a safe, containing space to allow the healing to occur.

Instructions for bringing the session to a close will depend on whether the soul fragment/part is ready to be integrated or not.

If more time is required then say:

'I would like to thank the soul fragment/part (which by now may have a name so use this instead) for joining us today and being brave in sharing its experiences. It would be really beneficial if we can meet again to continue this work and healing. Until then, I invite you to go back through the door that you first entered, wishing you well and I look forward to meeting you again.'

Ask the client to let you know when the soul fragment/part has left. Then follow the instructions for closing down the session provided below.

When you have permission for the client and their soul fragment or part to be integrated then you can say:

'I would like you to imagine sitting next to the soul fragment/part (if this part has a name, then use this instead). As you are sitting next to each other, I would like you to connect with the energy field or aura around each of you. As you do this, notice how the energy fields and auras start to merge. Keep allowing this to happen as the auras get more and more integrated until you are just one.'

(Pause)

Allow a few moments for this to happen and then ask the client to let you know when the energy fields or auras have completely integrated. Once integrated say to the client:

'Take a few slow deep breaths as you connect with this integrated part.'

Closing down the session

Regardless of whether the soul fragment/part has been integrated or not, the same procedure is used to close down the session by saying:

'I invite you to start bringing your awareness to the movement of the breath into and out of your body.'

(Pause)

'When you are ready, stand up and move towards the door that you initially entered, opening it up and stepping into the light, airy hallway. Then start to walk towards the front door of your house and open it up, stepping out into your garden and closing the front door behind. Take a few slow breaths of fresh air and connect with your senses as you notice with your surroundings in the garden.'

(Pause)

'Now start to walk down the pathway that leads from your house to the garden gate, taking in the surrounding scenery. When you arrive at the gate, open it up and step through, closing the gate behind you.'

(Pause)

'I would like you to start wiggling your fingers and toes, notice the surface of what you are sitting on and gently start opening up your eyes into the room you are in and back into the session with me today.'

Make sure you leave enough time for a debrief and ensure your client in grounded, using any of the resources that you have taught your client. You could also identify a positive statement by asking them what the most important positive or meaningful aspect of the session and install this with short slow BLS. Examples include:

- I am learning to understand myself better.
- I am learning to heal myself.
- I am learning to live a heart led and authentic life.
- I have all the strength I need within.
- I am learning to feel more integrated and whole.
- I have everything I need within.

Rebirthing procedure

Rebirthing is a technique used in several different alternative therapies including breathwork, as it is widely acknowledged that many traumas can be experienced during the birthing process. MacLean (2003) described three adult case studies where she used EMDR in a transpersonal way to help heal pre/perinatal trauma. O'Shea (2009) developed an Early Trauma Protocol and McGoldrick developed a preverbal AI-EMDR Protocol (©EMDR Insight, 2024) which you may like to experiment with.

The Rebirthing procedure described below has some similarities to the process in the EMDR future template where clients are invited to imagine playing a video to move through a period of time. In this situation the client is invited to imagine playing a video through their gestational journey. The video starts at a suitable positive place before the client experienced any distress or trauma, for example, the moment before incarnating, or the moment they felt their essence or soul enter their physical body in this incarnation. The client is then asked to notice any stage where there is some distress or negative affect, stop the video and process the distress using BLS. It enables a person to work through the trauma and have a different experience, processing and releasing any negative somatic or emotionally held sensations that have been blocked or repressed. It is something that I naturally did many years ago during a self-meditation as I was still holding on to the knowledge and feelings (some of them projected) that my birth had been traumatic for my mother; I was a very large baby, weighing 11 lbs! During this meditation, I connected with my divine essence, soul and spiritual resource team to guide me through the gestational phase. I imagined my Wise Self receiving and welcoming my baby self when born, holding and greeting her in a warm embrace using the loving eyes technique and creating a new co-construction of the narrative for my baby self. I found this to be a very powerful exercise.

It was when I was working with more complex cases, where traumas and attachment difficulties were apparent from birth, that I thought about trying a similar exercise with my clients. It is extremely helpful when there appears to be a disconnect between clients and their essence or soul from a very young age. I have worked with a number of clients where it was apparent that they dissociated in utero. I have also had a few clients become aware that they were a twin in utero but that their twin did not survive. In such instances, and if appropriate, you could discuss with your client whether they would like their twin's essence to become part of their spiritual support team moving forwards.

Instructions for rebirthing procedure

Set up the beginning of the session by following the initial four steps in the soul level section described earlier. Ask the client who they would like to act as their chosen midwife to deliver their younger baby self. This could be one of their nurturing, protective or wise figures, a spiritual figure, their Wise Self or someone else that has a positive and special significance for them. Make sure you have also identified and tested out a preferred BLS that the client can use at moments where they notice any distress, so that they can process any negative affect that arises. Also remember to show the client the stop signal.

You have the option of starting from different points of time so discuss what resonates for your client, amending the instructions below to take this into account. Possible options include, but are not exclusive to:

- The moment when they felt completely at one with the Divine Source (or source of healing light, spiritual home or any resource that resonates for the client).
- The moment they decided to incarnate into this lifetime from their spiritual home.
- The moment that their essence or soul decided to enter their physical body in utero in this lifetime, with a heart full of divine unconditional love.

Having chosen a suitable positive starting point, say:

'I would like you to connect with the moment when (choose the option below that links with their chosen starting point):

- *You were completely at one with the Divine Source (or source of healing light, spiritual home or resource that resonates for the client).*
- *You were still residing in your spiritual home and decided to incarnate.*
- *Your essence or soul decided to enter your physical body in utero in this lifetime, with a heart full of divine unconditional love.*

Remember you are completely in charge and can pause or stop at any stage. Imagine playing the video as you start to progress into the gestational period of this current incarnation. Any moments where you notice feeling distressing sensations, emotions or beliefs then let me know.'

After a few minutes, if the client has not asked to stop, ask them to pause the video and let you know what they noticed. If the feedback is positive, invite them to continue with the video, reminding them to let you know of any moments where they feel distressing sensations or emotions, negative beliefs or challenges. If something difficult or uncomfortable arises, ask the client to put the video on pause, briefly describe what they are noticing and apply some BLS to process through the discomfort. Once all the discomfort or distress has been processed ask them to continue on with the video, letting you know if any further discomfort or distress surfaces and if so, pause the video and apply some BLS until this discomfort has been processed.

If the client appears or reports feeling disconnected or dissociative, stop the exercise and support the client to ground themselves in the session. Once grounded and if they are wishing to continue, ask them to rewind the video to the moment just before they felt dissociative and ask them to bring in additional support such as a circle or bubble of protection from the Divine. Invite them to connect with any of their guides and spiritual support team that will also keep them safe from any harm. Once they have all the additional support in place, ask them to press play on their video and continue as before. It is a good idea to check with them at various intervals what they are noticing so that you can make sure they stay on track.

Continue with this process until they are ready to be born, processing any disturbance along the way with BLS. When they signal that they are ready to be born, make sure their chosen midwife is present to assist with the process.

Once born, ask your client to notice what they feel. If there is any negative affect, process this with some BLS. You can always suggest their chosen midwife look them in the eyes, if this feels comfortable to do so, and let them know how beautiful, loved, special and divinely protected they are. If their Wise Self has been the midwife, then you can then ask the client if they would like to integrate their baby self with their Wise Self as follows:

'I would like you to connect with the aura around your baby self and you representing your Wise Self. As you do this, notice how the energy fields and auras around you both start to merge. Keep allowing this to happen as the auras get more and more integrated until you are just one. Take a few slow deep breaths as you integrate with your baby self.'

When finishing the session, I would ask the client what has been the most positive or meaningful part that they can take away from this exercise, obtaining a positive affirmation or cognition that can be installed. Examples include:

- I have a heart full of love and divine light.
- I am wanted.
- I am loveable.
- I am worthy of love and support.
- I have all the divine support and protection I need.

Following the session, I would encourage the client to try and connect with their baby self each day to deepen the bond between them.

Remember to use your intuition during this work. You can link any of the questions and ideas discussed in the previous soul level healing section to the rebirthing procedure if it feels appropriate. For example, if the client's starting point was when they felt connected to their spiritual home before incarnating, they may find it helpful to explore some of the reasons why their soul decided to incarnate, what support is available to them, what role various other souls have in their life, including what are the lessons they are here to teach, learn or heal from these relationships. This information may assist them during the rebirthing process.

Case example: Susan and rebirthing procedure

Susan engaged with me having previously tried EMDR with several different clinicians but said that EMDR was not working for her; she had kept getting stuck, going blank and felt there was some unconscious block. During the initial appointment, it was apparent that Susan had a complex history. She spent her first six months in foster care before being adopted. Having had many years of therapy, she was still triggered by various past traumas and current interactions with others. Susan was a therapist herself and was using self-care techniques, but despite her self-awareness and self-compassion she said she had not been able to rid herself of some unpleasant physical reactions (often feelings of fear) that occurred in relation to certain family members and past memories. Susan said that she was open to spirituality but that it was a new area for her. She believed in a soul and was open to the idea of reincarnation. We discussed energies, triggers and mirrors and that she may have absorbed a multitude of projections from others throughout her life, including deep shame. Susan's core NCs included 'I don't matter,' 'I am bad,' 'I am invisible' with a repeated theme of being significantly rejected by others. She had watched the recorded online workshops and we were able to explore HLP and possible life lessons. One theme that kept emerging was 'independence' with a fear of living or speaking her true self. Susan often identified a pain in her throat, consistent with a block in her throat chakra, which was stopping her speaking her truth. Only once had she managed to walk away from someone and exert her independence, most other times in her life this had been very challenging to do. I sensed when we connected that Susan had learnt to dissociate very early in her life and I provided a formulation which incorporated concepts of HLP as well as the possibility of early dissociation. At the beginning, Susan was confident that she was not dissociative but was able to keep an open mind to the possibility. Intuitively I was sensing that we needed to start work in utero and asked whether we could try a rebirthing technique that I was trialling, to which she agreed as she was familiar with part work.

The initial part of the session involved Susan connecting her heart with the Divine Source and Mother Earth. Susan's starting point was the moment her essence entered into her physical body in utero. She connected with an image of the tiniest growth and a feeling that it wasn't possible; she was unwanted and knew what was to come. I therefore asked her to float back to the moment when she was completely at one with the Divine Source and she reported feeling emotional, all-perfect and wonderful. I then asked her to notice what happened next during the gestational period as she played the video, letting me know any moment where she felt some difficult emotions arise. Within six weeks of being in utero she connected with a knowing and feeling which was when her birth mother found out she was pregnant. Susan felt energy coming into her body, sadness, and a sense of wishing from her parents that she wasn't there. I asked her to notice that and start the BLS and she began to cry. She then said:

'I lose everything.'

The image disappeared, she was struggling to connect and this was the first moment where I believed she learnt to dissociate in life.

I guided Susan back to a time before she dissociated and we put some divine protection around her only letting in positive experiences and energy. She was then able to start running the video again. Below is the feedback that Susan provided during the times when I asked her to pause the video and any interweaves I used are shown after the word 'therapist.'

- *It's completely different this time. The baby is growing inside my birth mother. My birth mother knows she is pregnant and is sad as she knows my birth father doesn't want the baby but the baby is completely protected.*
- *The baby is big enough to be born. The birth father is dominant, the birth mother is passive. All the energy on the outside is negative and mostly from him.*

Therapist: Imagine you as your Wise Self now taking the role of the midwife.

- *(Tears). I am born and all wrapped up. I'm looking lovely.*

Therapist: If it feels comfortable to do so, are you able to look into the eyes of your younger self and send her love?

- *(Tears). Mission accomplished.*

To complete the session, I invited Susan to imagine her baby self and Wise Self's auras merging and integrating which she was able to do successfully.

This was a beautiful session for Susan and humbling for me to witness too. Susan was then able to work on various traumas using the standard EMDR protocol in proceeding sessions. At first, we did very short BLS sets, just dipping in to the memories briefly, shortening the length of BLS sets using Jim Knipe's CIPOS approach (Constant Installation of Present Orientation and Safety, Knipe, 2015) so that we could just dip in to the memory for five seconds and then build this up to ten seconds over the course of the session. This helped build up Susan's confidence in using EMDR and reconstruct her belief that she could process using EMDR. There were times during the first EMDR processing session when she didn't connect to anything but we continued, helping to clear the belief that she was not doing it as well as she should. With encouragement, she managed to keep going and process through this block as it had been part of her lived experience and she was soon able to process with much longer sets and start believing 'I can do this and I will be alright.' At the end of the next session's processing, which was incomplete, the most important meaning for her to take away from the processing had changed to 'I can do this, I am doing this!' In our third and final EMDR processing session, Susan worked through a difficult situation with some peers and at the end of the processing her positive or preferred cognition (PC) was 'I have an infinite source of love and light within me.'

EMDR attachment narratives incorporating a spiritual approach

Narrative EMDR was initially developed by Joan Lovett (Lovett, 1999, 2015) and is now widely recognised as an effective tool for very young children or those who are adopted, fostered or selective mute (Logie et al., 2020). The narrative is often used in the EMDR preparation stage and is sometimes all that is required to process traumas. I have also found it to be a powerful technique for adolescents as well as adults where there is a complex history of attachment difficulties and trauma. I developed a generic narrative for this client group to provide a gentler initial formulation, without detailing the specific traumas too early on which may overwhelm the person and result in dissociation. For this latter group, narrative EMDR can often help identify more specific memories to be processed once the story has been read.

Example of EMDR narrative for adolescent/adult

'I would like to share a story with you and it has a good ending. If you would like to stop at any stage then just raise your hand (show stop signal).

Once upon a time there was a beautiful person who had a big heart with so much love in it. When their spirit/essence entered this lifetime, their heart and soul were full of pure divine love and light. They managed to do many things in their life, perhaps this included going to school, maybe getting a job, playing different sports, being with other people or being creative.

As with all people, some things in life went well and some things in life were difficult and hard to understand. What was difficult and hard to understand was that when this person was born and just a little person, the people caring for them (this could have been their own parents or carers) didn't have the resources and skills to look after them in the way that all babies and young children need in order to form healthy attachments. Some of the difficult things that happened to this little person may have included being ignored or left alone for long periods of time, not given food when they were hungry, not had their nappies changed regularly or given clean clothes to wear. Maybe hurtful things were said or done to them and they may have witnessed lots of fighting, shout-ing or violence or abuse between other people or adults or other types of bad behaviour.

When these difficult experiences happened, it made the young person have lots of uncomfortable feelings in their body. This may have included feeling difficult emotions such as anxious, scared, sad, upset and angry too. Sometimes they may have felt uncomfortable physical feelings, including weakness in their legs or a tightness in their chest or a sick feeling, like a knot in their tummy. The little person was a sensitive soul and without consciously realising it, they may have absorbed many projections from other people in their life. Maybe they did this because they believed that it would help the other people feel better, or maybe they hadn't learnt how to protect their own energies and divine essence. As they absorbed the difficult negative energies, beliefs and sensations from other people, this made their own energy field feel saturated like a sponge. The young person didn't have anyone around to help them manage all the difficult energies or help them understand why all these painful experiences were happening. They had to figure this out themselves and one way they did this was to own all of these projections, maybe believing that it must be their fault or that they must be bad, unlovable, insignificant, didn't matter, were not good enough or unworthy. This may have made them feel tough emotions such as shame, guilt, loneliness, depression, anxiety or despair or experience difficult physical sensations. They also found it very hard to know how to trust others in their lives, especially adults, but also themselves.

The little person had to find their own way of managing all the horrible feelings in their body, so they decided to block them all out and disconnect from ANY emotions and physical feelings, including the good ones. This seemed to help a bit, so they carried on blocking and disconnecting what they were feeling. However, they were not able to block out the negative beliefs and these become stronger and stronger as time went on.

As the little person grew up, they may have found it difficult to make or keep friends, concentrate or remember what they were learning at school, and they may have been quite vulnerable at times and got into some trouble with other people or in different situations.

One day, they heard a person called a therapist read a story about similar things that had happened to other people when they had been younger. The story helped them to realise that they were not alone and that the feelings and thoughts that they had about themselves were because of the tough and traumatic experiences that had happened to them in their life. The story helped them to understand that the bad stuff that had happened was not their fault or that they had failed in anyway; it was actually because the people looking after them at the time just hadn't learnt the skills to manage their own feelings or negative beliefs or how to look after children. Perhaps this was because bad things had also happened to these adults in their life, which possibly meant that these adults may never have had a role model in their life or been shown how to bring children up in a safe, loving and calm environment. They realised that this was not an excuse for what had happened to them but it just helped them to understand that it was the adult's responsibility for providing a safe, loving and caring environment; no child, whatever the circumstances, deserves to be treated in a bad, neglectful, abusive or harmful way. They also learnt that it is not their responsibility to absorb difficult energies from those around them, even if they think it might help other people.

The story helped the person learn that the way they had shut down their emotions and physical feelings when they were little and growing up was something called dissociation. They were told that this was a survival technique which helped keep them alive and get through all the tough and traumatic times. However, they were also taught that when they started living in a safer environment, they didn't need to dissociate anymore, as this was stopping them forming new, healthier relationships and positive experiences with people. They started to learn how to safely connect to more positive feelings, beliefs and emotions in their body. This helped them to feel calmer, happier and stronger.

The person may also have needed to get some extra support to help them process the traumas they had been through so that these didn't impact on them anymore. They found a way of asking for help from trusted adults or friends (or maybe even teachers or health care professionals) in their life to support them to find the right person who could do this work safely with them. They were shown how to understand themselves as an energetic being and learn techniques for how to protect and clear their own energies on a regular basis as part of their ongoing self-care. They learnt how to form a positive relationship with their heart and soul and connect with this regularly to start discovering and trusting their own truth and authenticity. They also learnt how to connect with beautiful, positive energies in their life that were more in resonance with their own. This may have been with certain loving people, being in nature or in certain environments and situations. As they embraced this, their self-worth, self-love and respect for themselves deepened as they recognised they have a choice in how they could live their lives. Maybe they also learnt how to connect or reconnect with a bigger energy field outside of them which was full of unconditional and infinite divine love. This may have included connecting with a universal support team including guides, teachers, ancestors, ascended masters, angels, God, Buddha, Mohammed or whatever resonated with their own beliefs and inner truth. This helped the person start learning to believe they were lovable, good enough, that they mattered, were worthwhile and blameless to past experiences and that they were deserving of being in alignment with their true divine essence. As they learnt how to do this more and more on a regular basis, the light and divine essence that was always within them began to grow stronger and brighter each day.

The person began to feel proud of themselves and they became braver and braver. They started to realise that whatever tough challenges and experiences they had, they also had the inner strength and courage to overcome these and start living a healthier life. They were also able to believe that they really had been born with such a beautiful big heart and soul or essence, which had so much love in it, and that no-one or nothing could or would ever change this. They just had to connect with their heart regularly which gave them the strength and courage they needed to succeed in whatever they chose to do in their life. They also realised that even during times when they felt doubt or loneliness or tough feelings or beliefs in their life, they were never alone; they were always supported universally and always had an infinite and unbreakable connection with their chosen Divine Source.

The End'

If I read the generic narrative as part of the formulation and have not yet explained about EMDR then I do not use BLS. However, if I introduce the generic narrative (or an amended version that is more specific to the client's history) as part of the preparation stage of EMDR and we have discussed EMDR and checked appropriate BLS, then I use BLS continuously throughout the story as it may deepen the experience. Please tweak and amend the narrative according to your clients' spiritual beliefs.

When I read the story, I monitor how the client responds to various sections of the story, looking out for feedback (nonverbal or energetic) about specific areas that may be resonating more than others. At the end of the story, I will ask the client what they think of the story and ask whether there is anything they feel needs changing or adding.

Often the client will say 'did you write that about me?' because many aspects of the story will resonate. We may then gently explore what they are feeling from having heard the story. The narrative often helps sow the seeds for subsequent sessions, including resourcing, possible ego state, part work or inner child work and helps the client begin to have a kinder, more compassionate understanding of themselves and their earlier life experiences.

Possible amendments include:

- If they are fairly new to spiritual concepts then you could change some of the wording to say, 'they were open to learning about the possibility that they could connect to a universal support' or 'they were open to learning to believe that they were born with a heart full of love and light.'
- 'They were learning to understand themselves as an energy body.'
- If they don't believe in incarnation, then you could say 'the moment when their heart started beating in utero, it was completely full of the love and light.'

Working with refugees

I haven't worked directly with refugees but have supervised EMDR colleagues, especially those working with children and adolescents. For several years, I supervised a lovely EMDR practitioner in a child and adolescent mental health service (CAMHS) team whose main caseload was working with refugees from Afghanistan and often her sessions were online with the support of an interpreter. Whilst she was a skilled therapist, she sometimes found it hard to make significant positive changes with this client group due to language barriers, the devastating traumas they had experienced and the isolation that many felt having been separated from their families, friends and country. Over time, I worked on helping the therapist to connect more from an energetic perspective with her clients. It felt intuitively important that whilst the situation seemed bleak, there was a great deal of hope that could come from introducing various spiritual resources where appropriate. The New Extended Light Stream was often a huge success, as well as using various aromatherapy oils, crystals, etc. to help the client to self-soothe. The therapist also started introducing an EMDR narrative, creating a very simple version of the client's experience that wouldn't overwhelm them. Often, much of the client's history remained unknown because they were too traumatised and dissociative to share their experience. The narrative was a way of introducing aspects of the EMDR processing (NC, PC, emotions, body location) to bring about positive change. A key part of the story included the idea of an invisible and infinite cord between the client's heart and their family or loved ones, despite being so far apart, or at times not knowing whether they were still alive. If appropriate, and often it was, the story would include helping the client to connect in their heart with aspects of their faith and use this as a means to strengthen themselves at any time in order not to feel so alone or vulnerable. The therapist began to have a huge success with the EMDR narrative and often it was enough to bring about significant change in different areas of the clients' life including eating, sleeping, learning at school and interactions with others. Occasionally it enabled the client to share more detail of specific traumas and if this was the case either the EMDR narrative was adapted to take these into account or the EMDR standard protocol was used.

Below is a general framework of a story that can be adapted according to your client's faith, gender, culture, beliefs, etc. It can be used as a template for any person who may have experienced having to leave their own country due to difficult circumstances. Each client's experiences will be different so adapt according to what you know and what is appropriate and I have used 'the boy' just to provide an example, but please alter accordingly to fit with your client and their chosen gender identification. As a general rule of thumb, please start simply. You can always add aspects to the story over sessions but it is important not to overwhelm the client and prioritise maintaining a good, safe therapeutic relationship.

Example of an EMDR narrative for a refugee

'This is a story that has a good ending. If you would like to stop at any stage then just raise your hand (show stop signal).

Once upon a time a beautiful boy was born. Just like everyone else in the world, this boy had some things in his life that were lucky and some things that were difficult and hard to understand. One lucky thing was that he was born a healthy and lovable baby with a heart full of beautiful love and light. Just like all babies, he deserved to be loved, nurtured, cared for, and kept safe. As the boy grew, he was funny, good at sports, loved drama and cooking and playing with his friends.

What was difficult and hard to understand was that the boy was growing up in a country where lots of people were fighting and at war with each other. This made the boy feel scared inside and he believed he wasn't safe and was in *danger. Maybe he saw some difficult things happen to his family or friends or maybe things happened to him that were distressing.*

When the boy was older, he had to suddenly leave his country, family and friends. Maybe he didn't have time to say goodbye to the people he loved and this could have made him feel very sad and lonely in his body and worried about whether he would ever be able to see any of them again. He may have worried about what happened to the people who stayed behind in his country where the fighting was happening.

The boy had experienced some really tough challenges as he journeyed to a different country and at times he feared for his own safety. He continued to feel very alone, scared and anxious in his body. One day he arrived in a new country where everything was unfamiliar and he didn't know how to speak the language of this new country very well. He may have started living with a relative who had also come to this country and this may have been someone whom he didn't have a very close relationship.

When all of these difficult experiences happened, it made the boy have lots of uncomfortable feelings in his body. The boy had to find his own way of managing all the horrible feelings in his body so he decided to block them all out and disconnect from ANY emotions and physical feelings, including the good ones. This seemed to help a bit so he carried on blocking and disconnecting what he was feeling. He may have shut himself away or stopped speaking very much to anyone around him, or he may have found it hard to sleep and eat because he was feeling so unhappy and alone.

The boy started going to a local school which was difficult as everything was unfamiliar. Some of the teachers were kind and tried to support him to settle in to his new environment. Some adults could see how hard things were for this boy and they found a person, called a therapist, who tried to help support the boy with the difficult experiences and challenges that he had gone through. Another person, called an interpreter, may have also been in these sessions to help translate what was being said by the therapist.

The therapist helped the boy to remember that he had always had a heart full of love and light. The boy was reminded that he had an infinite and unbreakable bond between his heart and everyone he loved and cared about, no matter where they lived in the world. The boy learnt that this unbreakable and infinite bond continued regardless of whether the person was still alive or whether they had died and he could connect and send love to them just by connecting in his heart. The boy also remembered that his faith was very important to him and that he was very much loved by this loving source (make specific to your client's belief system) *and that that this source of support and love and light was also infinite and unbreakable.*

The boy learnt that when he was feeling alone or scared, all he had to do was connect in his heart and with this loving source and feel the unconditional love and light flow into his body. This helped release the difficult feelings or beliefs that he had been experiencing and fill his body with the unconditional love and healing light. Practising this regularly helped the boy to feel stronger and stronger.

Soon the boy started feeling happier at school and started to do well in his lessons and make new friends. The boy also knew that even though he was not able to be with his family and friends from his own country at the moment, he could connect in his heart and send them love anytime wherever he was and that his family and friends would receive and feel this love. This helped the boy feel more settled and at peace in life.

The End'

EMDR narratives for younger children

This is generally covered very well in Lovett and Logie et al.'s books so there are not many changes I would recommend. The examples provided usually start with the notion that the child was born lovable, regardless or not of whether they were born into a supportive family. I would start the narrative with:

'The child was born with a heart full of love,'

as this helps introduce the idea of an energetic heart connection. Depending on the age of the child and circumstances, I might include the notion of the unbreakable, infinite cord from their heart to someone else's if appropriate, or ideas could include the child learning that no matter what anyone did or said to them, they learnt to believe their heart was always full of infinite love.

Summary

- Clients who present with complex presentations often need more preparation and resource work before starting the EMDR processing. Some of the techniques to assist with this includes part and inner child work. Part work can assist clients to form a deeper healing heart and soul level connection with their inner child.
- It is important for therapists to consciously be working at coming into alignment with their own heart and soul in order to carry out soul part work.
- Using the recommended four initial steps before starting soul level work enables both client and therapist to establish a safe, containing, energetic environment.
- Clients can be assisted to find a safe and protected place in order to connect with their spiritual home and gain wisdom and support that will assist them on their spiritual journey.
- Clients can be assisted to find a safe and protected place in order to reclaim lost soul parts or fragments.
- A rebirthing procedure is useful when the client may have experienced trauma when incarnating, in utero or during the birthing process.
- EMDR narratives can be used to provide a formulation to clients about the attachment and trauma difficulties they have experienced that take into

account an energy perspective. These can be adapted to incorporate the clients' spiritual beliefs. The narratives can also be used in the preparation stages of EMDR, which provides a gentle introduction into EMDR therapy and can then lead to processing on the more specific traumas.

- EMDR narratives can be adapted and provide a valuable tool when working with different client populations and spiritual beliefs, for example, when working with refugees.

Chapter 12

EMDR Phase 3

Assessment

'I close my eyes in order to see.'

Paul Gauguin

By the time you arrive at the assessment phase of EMDR therapy, you should hopefully have prepared yourself energetically before the session and set up the surroundings to create a safe, supportive space. Remember the significance of the spiritual resonance and connection with your client. Are your energies and alignment conducive to providing the best chance of multi-dimensional healing? Are you regulating your breathing, connecting with your heart space and directing that positive healing energy towards your client? Ideally, your client should also have the spiritual and energy resources they need to self-soothe and be practising this regularly.

The assessment phase has two main purposes. The first is to access the main areas of the maladaptive memory network. The second is to determine baseline measures for the target memory which act as the point of reference for the proceeding phases of EMDR therapy to monitor progress. Some EMDR therapists are much more willing to start processing quicker than others, regardless of the client's complexity, so there are different schools of thought about time required to spend in the preparation phase. Four key areas that help determine a client's readiness for processing include:

- Ability to form a therapeutic relationship, as well as motivation and level of insight.
- Ability to self-soothe or cope with high levels of affect.
- Current level of risk, including whether they are actively self-harming or highly dependent on substance use.
- Current level of functioning. Are they able to access support from family, friends, pets, work, school or community or are they living in complete isolation?

From a spiritual perspective, my personal view is that teaching your client resources and coping strategies is an essential part of the journey regardless of

DOI: 10.4324/9781003509646-15

whether or not you go on to use EMDR. A spiritual journey can be exceptionally challenging and brutal at times as one accesses areas in life that are no longer in alignment with one's authenticity. Therefore, learning the techniques to work through and manage these challenges is crucial. Resources not only prepare clients for EMDR, but also teach them essential self-care strategies that they can continue to use beyond EMDR sessions, softening the impact of any future difficulties or energetic shifts.

I tend to view EMDR as the icing on the cake. If I prepare the client sufficiently, including psychoeducation, mindfulness and various resource and coping strategies and have established a strong spiritual resonance and healthy positive energetic space in sessions, then my clinical observation is that processing tends to be smoother, sometimes faster and fewer interweaves are required. I would also only ever use HLP interweaves and ideas (including differentiating between the ego and heart, life lessons and being the observer) if I have taught the client HLP before we start processing, otherwise the client is unlikely to know what I am referring to and this will confuse them.

R. Shapiro (2009) described using the standard protocol in her chapter on working with religious-spiritual attuned clients. The standard or modified protocol can be applied when using HLP-informed EMDR unless there is clinical justification that a different protocol may be required for example, addiction, phobia, pain, prolonged grief protocols, etc. (F. Shapiro, 2018). Accessing the affect is the key goal during the assessment phase (Shapiro, 2018) and there is much more emphasis nowadays on different ways to do this for more complex presentations, including using the 'Tip of the Finger' technique (Gonzalez, Mosquera & Fisher, 2012).

It is important at the beginning of the assessment phase to check with your client what type of BLS fits with their belief system or is most comfortable for them. For example, some cultures may see eye movements as witchcraft (Mbazzi et al., 2021). Some may not be comfortable with being touched, so different forms of tactile BLS can be offered, for example, the client can tap their own body at a suitable, safe place, engage with ritualistic movements that align with their cultural and spiritual beliefs, or tap a table or floor with their feet. Perhaps an advantage about using other forms of BLS to eye movements is that the client, where clinically safe to do so, can close their eyes and go within and access their 'inner wisdom.' I was never able to use eye movements with clients when I first trained due to physical injuries, and whilst new technology has since developed that can facilitate eye movements, I rarely use this unless it is the client's preference. I have never found this to be a hindrance or disadvantage to my EMDR sessions. It is also not unusual for me to observe clients' eyes naturally move from side to side under closed eyelids during processing.

Make sure that you have established a suitable stop signal with the client. Whilst I am aware that some EMDR clinicians do not advocate the necessity of ever teaching clients a stop signal because they interpret its use as avoidance, from a trauma perspective, allowing your clients to know that they have the control to stop the processing at any stage can be very empowering. Clients may have had experiences where their nervous systems shut down and froze, leaving them with a sense of powerless in their traumas, unable to run away or stop the trauma or abuse from happening. Most clients do not need to use the stop signal, but knowing it is there is healing in itself and gives them a sense of mastery. Again, cultural adaptations may be required, especially if the hand signal is interpreted as rude or offensive. In such cases, it is important to check in with the client more frequently to make sure they are comfortable to continue during the processing (Mbazzi et al., 2021).

During the assessment phase, I have personally found that ascertaining the negative cognition (NC) provides information that can help identify or confirm the blocks and restrictions from a HLP perspective, as well as offer some insight or confirmation into what life lessons may be occurring for an individual. It can also provide potential guidance of past life themes that may still be played out including possible soul level blocks and restrictions, for example, a sense of peril that they may be found out or persecuted, believing they are to blame, unlovable, undeserving, unworthy, not trusting others which may have actually been their soul's experience in past incarnations. In addition, whilst I have experimented with not always ascertaining the NC when trying different protocols, for me, I notice I am more able to fully connect with the client and keep them on track when I do have this information. Again, this is a personal choice and I respect that others may have a different perspective.

Some cultures experience challenging situations as a group rather than individually (Mbazzi et al., 2021), so the NC and PC may need to be more flexible and take this into account, for example,

Negative Cognition (NC)	Positive/Preferred Cognition (PC)
• We are cursed	We are healed or cleansed.
• We failed	We achieved, succeeded or are a success.
• We are not safe	We are safe now.

You may also need to change the wording of NC to 'bad' thoughts and PC as 'good' or 'blessed' thoughts.

Chakras and associated body locations

I mentioned the chakras earlier in this book and for those of you that are familiar with them, you will be aware that the chakras represent various energy centres in the body corresponding to specific nerve bundles and internal organs. Some believe that chakras represent psychic centres of transformation, enabling a person to move towards enlightenment (Johari, 2000). For each of the seven main chakras in the physical body, there may be associated names and specific locations within the body, colour, shape, sound, aspects, etc. Chakras can become blocked and not function very well when a person has experienced trauma. For simplicity's sake, I am illustrating the key characteristics that are generally associated with chakras.

- **Root chakra**: Representing our foundation and located at the base of the spine giving a sense of being grounded. Linked to core survival, including areas such as finances, independence, money and food. When blocked, a person may feel threatened, unsafe, ungrounded and disconnected from their environment.
- **Sacral chakra**: Representing how we relate to our emotions, emotions of others as well as our centre of creativity, sexuality and reproduction. Located in the lower abdomen about two inches below the navel. Linked to areas of abundance, well-being, pleasure and sexuality. When blocked, a person may have issues in the areas of abundance, sexual intimacy, creativity and connecting emotionally with others as well as themselves.
- **Solar plexus chakra**: Representing how a person is confident, in control of their life and able to freely express their true self. Located in the upper abdomen in the stomach area. Linked to areas of self-worth, self-confidence and self-esteem. When blocked, a person may struggle with lack of control, power or empowerment and feel overwhelming amounts of anxiety, self-doubt and shame.
- **Heart chakra**: This represents the meeting point of the lower three chakras (associated with materiality) and upper three chakras (associated with spirituality) and is the centre of unconditional love, joy and inner peace and represents our ability to give and receive love. It is located in the centre of the chest just above the physical heart structure. When blocked, a person may struggle to fully open themselves up to others, receive as well as give unconditional love or have self-love.
- **Throat chakra**: Representing a person's ability to communicate their truth, authenticity and personal loving power. It is located in the throat area of the physical body. When blocked, a person may have issues in the areas of speaking their truth and self-expression.
- **Third eye chakra**: Representing a person's ability to see the bigger picture (spiritually) and connect with their intuition. Located in the forehead between the eyes. When blocked, a person may have issues in the areas of vision and intuitive skills.
- **Crown chakra**: This is the highest chakra in the physical body and represents a person's ability to be full connected spiritually. Situated at the crown of the head and when fully open and clear, it enables a person to connect with a higher consciousness. When blocked, a person may have issues in the areas of spirituality, deeper meaning and spiritual connection in their life.

From a spiritual and energetic perspective, I hold a level of curiosity about where the client locates their distress in their physical body as established in the location of body sensation (BS) question. For example, it is not uncommon in traumas for clients who have struggled to speak their truth or be heard to have associated blocks in their throat chakra and locate their distress around their throat, jaw and shoulders. Clients who struggle with anxiety may often locate their distress around the solar plexus or sacral chakras. Those who are struggling with self-love or receiving love in relationships may have blocks around their heart chakra. I think the important point is to retain a level of curiosity but without over-analysing as you may be wrong. However, it can sometimes provide clarification of what you might be noticing energetically or intuitively and could offer some guidance if any interweaves are required during processing, as discussed in the next chapter. I would only discuss chakras with clients who are familiar or open to the possibility of energy centres.

Soul level work

This was mentioned in the previous chapter, but I include it once again as a reminder to illustrate the different steps you can take if intentionally deciding to work at a soul level. If you and your client have decided to complete some soul level EMDR processing, then it is important to make sure you have agreement with the client's soul that they are willing to engage in this healing. Making it explicit brings it into the client's conscious awareness. Also, it is imperative that your client has the awareness, motivation, capacity, internal and external resources to be able to undertake soul level work. Chapter 15 outlines clinical presentations where it would *not* be suitable.

These are the steps that I would recommend considering when working at a soul level to incorporate at the beginning of the assessment phase, before proceeding with exploring the questions related to the target or memory you have decided to work on.

1   Ask for agreement from the client and their soul/essence to work on the presenting trauma.
2   Create a protective energetic space for you and your client. This may be something pertinent to them or connecting with the Divine Source and asking for a protective barrier to surround and your client. You may choose to use one of the protection examples provided in Chapters 2 and 10.
3   Check that all parts of the client are happy to work on the trauma. If not, then invite those parts that are not willing to participate to go to their safe/peaceful/calm/sacred place where they can rest until the session has been completed.
4   Here are some additional stages which you can support your client to do:

- Connect with the quantum field where all possibilities exist.
- Connect with spiritual resource teams which may include spiritual, nurturing, protective and wise figures, power animals etc.
- Connect with the breath and then bring the breath into the heart and soul area. You could use one of the scripts provided in Chapters 5 and 6.
- Imagine a healing cord or line flowing from their heart downwards through the body into Earth and anchoring itself deep into Mother Earth to feel grounded.
- Imagine a healing cord or line going from their heart, upwards through the top of the body and connecting with a place of choice (Divine, God, Buddha, Allah, Sun, Moon, particular healing realm, etc).
- If you are trained in Akashic Record healing then, with their permission, you could connect with their Akashic Records. Remember to close down the Akashic Records once the work is complete.

Next, ask the client (and you do this as well) to centre themselves in their heart and/or soul.

If you have already started the desensitisation phase but the client is getting blocked, feeling very disconnected from their soul or spiritual support, or struggling to hold a transpersonal or spiritual perspective to their difficulties, then it is advisable to pause further processing (close down the processing as an incomplete session) and return to focus on more preparation work using deeper soul work as discussed in the previous chapter.

Float/bridge-back to past lives

I am using the word floatback in this book as it is a term taught in most EMDR standard training courses, but the term can be rather confusing as it suggests clients are 'floating.' Perhaps a more grounding and relatable term is bridge-back (Parnell, 2007), so please just use whatever resonates for you and your clinical practice.

Clients may spontaneously float back to past lives with little guidance required, and this may happen when you are identifying a touchstone memory during the assessment phase or during processing. Below are some instructions of how to assist your client to float back to past lives during the assessment phase.

As part of the assessment phase:

Ask your client to connect with a memory or incident in this current lifetime that represents a situation which is keeping them stuck repeating ego cycles (memory A). This may be representing a soul level block and restriction. As they connect to the worst moment in that memory, ask your client to identify the associated NC, affect, or both, and where they notice it in their body. Then say:

'As you connect to the worst moment in this memory and the NC {insert their NC} and emotions {insert their emotions}, notice the sensations you feel in your body and allow your mind to float back to the earliest time when you have felt this way before. This may have been in this life or in previous lifetimes. Just let whatever arises to do so without judgement or criticism. Just allow whatever to happen to happen and let me know when you land somewhere.'

When the client informs you that they have connected with a memory (memory B), this will now be your starting point and point of reference that you will return to during the processing or following an incomplete session. If the client has connected with another current lifetime memory or incident, you could repeat the instructions above to see whether they can float back any earlier, perhaps to a past life. You will know when you have arrived at the memory to work on as the client will not be able to connect with anything earlier in time.

Once you have the target memory (memory B), proceed with the assessment stage using the standard or modified protocol and start the BLS. The client may stay with that memory or connect with different memories from that lifetime or other lifetimes. Just let whatever happens happen, remaining out of the way as much as possible rather than asking too many questions (which is probably just your curiosity and ego!). Remember that the earliest memory (memory B) which you completed the assessment phase questions is the point of reference that you will come back to (i.e., original incident) when the client appears to have worked through material or various channels to a positive resolution.

Once memory B has been processed to completion, it is advisable to re-evaluate the first current memory before you did the floatback technique (memory A). You may still need to process memory A if there is distress still associated with it, but by now hopefully any feeder memories or blocks will have been removed.

Summary

- It is important to have established an energetically safe, containing environment with your client before commencing with the assessment phase.
- The four key areas to consider in determining whether your client is ready to proceed into the assessment phase include their ability to form a therapeutic relationship with you, their ability to self-soothe or manage high levels of affect, current level of risk and have some connection with the outside world.
- Some cultures may have NC and PC that refer to their place within their particular community, e.g., 'we' rather than 'I.'
- There are seven main chakras, known to represent energy centres, in the physical body.

- Holding a level of curiosity about the link between where the client is holding any distress in their body (BS) with an associated chakra can be informative and provide some guidance to suitable interweaves that may be required during processing.
- Those clients who are open to reincarnation can be guided to float back to a past lifetime when an underlying soul level block may have occurred that is still impacting on them in this current lifetime.

Chapter 13

EMDR Phase 4

Desensitisation

'The only really lasting beauty is the beauty of the heart.'

Rumi

You are now at the stage where your client is ready to start processing their target memory. I personally find it most beneficial when everything has already been set up and explained to the client at the beginning of the assessment phase, so that I can support the clients to move smoothly into processing, as often they will already be activated and in their material from the assessment questions. I have observed that with certain clients who are embracing and integrating their spiritual journey into many areas of their life, the processing can happen very intensely and rapidly. However, I urge any therapist to not interpret this too much and to let go of expectations. I have also noticed that when Light Language comes through, it can really facilitate the healing process in most cases, but I never plan to use this or see it as a way of accelerating or bypassing the processing, I just surrender and trust. Stay humble in your approach.

Working intuitively or energetically during desensitisation

As the processing flows and you are connected and aligned in your heart and with the Divine (or your preferred healing source), become aware of the soul whispers or 'knowings' that come through. Do you notice any physical changes in your body as your client processes certain areas or make comments about what has just come up for them? Are there thoughts that pop into your head or guidance as to a particular interweave that may be helpful if the client appears stuck? Are you feeling certain emotions or other physical sensations that the client may or may not be in touch with? Are there images or visions that appear to you? It really doesn't matter if none of this happens, but if it does, just stay as the observer and navigator, as it may be a sign or confirmation of what is happening for your client.

During processing, as well as each of the stages of the EMDR therapy, try to hold in mind the transference or energetic connection within the room. Be

DOI: 10.4324/9781003509646-16

aware of the mirror neurones and how this is impacting on you and your client emotionally, physically, spiritually and cognitively. What are the messages you are receiving or noticing within? Are they mirroring something back to you or triggering you in a way that is showing something that needs addressing or healing within yourself. If your client seems to be stuck, is this how you are also feeling in the session or is it reflecting back to you something in your life that you are feeling stuck with? Keep a check on your breathing, stature and any changes occurring within you, and as you stay regulated and within your window of tolerance, this will support your client to do the same energetically. Be prepared to find time to explore and heal your own material and triggers outside of your client's sessions.

Abreactions

If my client is having an abreaction, I will intuitively and mindfully connect with my breath to help with the energetic attunement and establish a calm pace in my breathing. Within a short period of time, I often notice that the client's breath starts to synchronise with mine, even when they have their eyes closed. We are dancing and flowing in the energetic space in the session. Sometimes, if a client is having a significant abreaction, I may be intuitively guided to provide some additional regulation through the energetic connection. This can sometimes be in the form of Light Language. Other times, I might centre more on my heart and increase the amount of love and healing from my heart and soul to theirs. If the client is using tactile or sound BLS, I may suggest we make eye contact if they are able to tolerate this, and I breath in and out with them as they are processing to help keep them grounded and connected. My voice is soft and present, offering a few reassuring words; *'that's it, I am here with you, you are doing really well'* and I observe their breath slowly come into sync with mine. All the time this is happening, I am intentionally connecting with them at a heart and soul level, sending love and healing energies.

Talkative clients

Some clients will be quite talkative during processing, despite having been told that only brief feedback is required. They may talk during the BLS or want to give you a lot of feedback in between sets. I have heard some EMDR clinicians talk about a 'ten-second rule,' suggesting that after ten seconds, interrupt the client to get them processing again. Whilst I agree that it is important to keep the flow of processing going, I am aware that there are clients who have had past experiences of never been heard or listened to. They may have been 'shut down' time and time again, so care needs to be given not to re-enact this in the session. The processing may be an opportunity for them to start learning to be heard, validated and speak their truth. Using your clinical judgement, intuition and awareness of the spiritual resonance between you and your client will support you in adopting a flexible approach and ascertaining the significance of their need to speak. It may be helping clear energy from their throat chakra that could have been blocked for many past lives, so allowing them to speak in itself is offering multi-dimensional healing. Sometimes for the very talkative clients, I let the BLS continue when they are speaking so that they are still processing during this time and when it feels a suitable moment, I may then say, 'just notice that.' This often guides the client to go within and they may naturally quieten down in a more reflective, peaceful way.

Interweaves

Interweaves are used when clients are stuck or looping during processing and are only taught in the latter parts of EMDR standard accredited trainings. The therapist first needs to grapple with the basics of EMDR and try different approaches if the client is stuck, for example, change in direction, speed of chosen BLS, float/bridge-back to touchstone memory and so forth. Interweaves are more likely to be used for complex clients who have significant histories of attachment difficulties or trauma and it is a technique that facilitates the client to get back on track with the processing so that they can access their adaptive network.

The therapist takes the role of the navigator, trusting the process, their client and their client's insights which can be really powerful and transformational. I personally believe that the most powerful interweaves are those that are intuitive and guided by the energetic and spiritual connection between myself, the client and the Divine. This process involves stepping away from egoic thoughts and fears and being completely aligned in my heart and soul. Dobo (2023) describes a similar process which he refers to as connecting with the 'inner genius' of oneself and the client.

Interweaves should, ideally, be used sparingly, allowing the client to have an internal experience and provide an opportunity to self-heal. However, there are times when the therapist does need to step in and offer some assistance to facilitate the client to get back on track. Interweaves generally fall into the categories of cognitive, visual, educational, imaginary or spiritual. The majority of interweaves taught on EMDR trainings fall into the first set of categories, so this section will focus on different types of spiritual interweaves.

Various spiritual interweaves have been described before (Parnell, 2008; Dent, 2020), which include helping the client to access spiritual guides, supporters, Divine Source, Wise Self or a larger universal or cosmic awareness that may resonate with them personally. Siegel (2017) described using 'cosmic' interweaves, which she explained as filling the therapeutic space with a divine presence or cosmic awareness, enabling her clients to connect to their higher selves, in order to facilitate a positive shift in their belief system.

More specific HLP informed interweaves can be applied if HLP has been discussed with the client previously in the preparation stages. This means they already understand the language and concepts you are referring to and can apply these ideas smoothly during the processing. For example, the client has some understanding of connecting with their heart and soul, being the observer and deciphering what the experience may be teaching them.

Examples of different HLP spiritual interweaves

These include:

1. **Listening to their heart and soul**: When a client appears stuck in egoic thinking during EMDR processing, before starting the next set of BLS ask them to either:

    'Move into your heart and/or soul and listen to what your heart and/or soul is trying to tell you.'

    'What is the message from your heart and/or soul?'

    'Connect with your heart.'

2. **Life lessons**: When the client appears stuck, ask them:

    'What do you think this challenge or situation is helping you to understand or experience?'

3. **Teaching, learning or healing**: similar to the life lessons, when a client is stuck in processing a difficult encounter with another person, then it may be helpful for you to ask your client:

    'What do you think this relationship or situation is trying to teach, learn or heal either for yourself or them?'

4. **Heart connection with another person**: if appropriate you could say:

    'Imagine an infinite, unbreakable cord running from your heart to another person (this could be someone that is deceased, someone they haven't seen or someone they are unsure whether is alive or not).'

5. **Energy interweave**: Ask your client to connect to their heart and say either:

    'Whose energy is this that you are feeling in your body?'

    'Is this your energy or someone else's?'

6. **Releasing energy**: If you felt that the client was struggling to release a difficult energy and was open to the Divine or another spiritual support then you can ask them to connect with their particular spiritual support and ask that this facilitates the clearing of the energy during the next BLS

set. If you have introduced the portal-clearing exercise in the preparation stages of EMDR, then you could bring this in. Invite your client to open the portal to facilitate the release of the energy through the portal so that it can be transmuted into love, light or divine energy. Then start the BLS. Remember to close the portal at the end of the session.

7. **Intergenerational and ancestral healing**: For those clients who have experienced a great deal of intergenerational or ancestral trauma and that is impacting or blocking their processing, you can invite your client to connect in their heart and/or soul and say:

'If this feels comfortable for you to do so, imagine sending a healing light and energy from your heart and/or soul down the ancestral or generational line. You could also imagine sending this healing light to any future generations too. You may also wish to connect with a Divine healing light and send this down the ancestral or generational line.'

You may need to do a longer set of BLS whilst this is happening.

8. **Healing past lives**: Similar to the ancestral or intergenerational healing, if the client is open to reincarnation and is aware of a soul level block or theme that has been running through many lifetimes, they can imagine sending healing love from their heart to all their previous and future lifetimes to clear this energy. You could ask your client:

'If this feels comfortable for you to do so, imagine sending a healing light and energy from your heart and/or soul to all the past lives that you have experienced. You could also imagine sending this healing light to any future versions of yourself too. You may also wish to connect with a Divine healing light and send to all past and future lifetimes or versions of yourself.'

You may need to do a longer set of BLS whilst this is happening.

9. **Clearing blocked chakras**: If a client is noticing tension or a block in one of their chakras, then you could provide suitable instructions for an action that they could now do in imagination, which they were unable to do at the time, to help release the block. An example is if the client is struggling to clear some tension around their throat, a possible interweave might be:

'If there was something that you wish you had said, but were unable to say at the time because it was unsafe to do so, can you say this now in your imagination? You can scream, shout or do whatever feels most comfortable as it is safe to do so now.'

Other possible ideas could be imagining running away from the trauma scene if there was a block in their base chakra, connecting with an infinite unbreakable cord of love from the Divine or another loving source if there was a block in their heart chakra, etc. Use your intuition and support the client to be creative and imaginative. Your client may need to move, shake part of their body or perform some other physical action to facilitate releasing any stuck energy.

Two handed interweave

One of my favourite interweaves is the two handed interweave by Shapiro (2005) which can be a really useful way of separating out two different conundrums, or identify what is good about holding on to something (emotion, belief, etc.) and what is good about letting it go. For example, if a client is oscillating between different thought processes, it can help separate them out by putting one thought process in the left hand, and the other in the right hand. It can also assist with supporting the client to identify what is good or meaningful about holding on to something (placed metaphorically in one hand) and what is good at letting something go (metaphorically placed in the other). Below are some examples of how to incorporate the idea of HLP using the two handed interweave. A few of these exercises were discussed in Chapters 4 and 6 but here is where you can add the BLS to facilitate processing.

1. When you or your client start to differentiate more easily between their ego and heart responses you could suggest:

    'Imagine placing what your ego is saying in one hand. Just let it rest there. Imagine in your other hand placing what your heart is saying, again allowing it to rest there. Just notice that,'
    then start the BLS.

2. If the client is struggling with two different scenarios (e.g., should they stay or leave a relationship or situation), you could ask them to first connect in their heart, then place one of the scenarios metaphorically into each hand. Ask them to stay connected with their heart and start the BLS, encouraging your client to allow whatever happens to happen.

3. If a client is noticing energy, emotions or beliefs in their system that they recognise is not theirs, then say:

    'Imagine in your left hand connecting with what is good about holding on to this energy, emotion or belief.'

Wait for a response before saying:

'Imagine in your right hand connecting with what is good about letting go of this energy, emotion or belief.'

Wait for a response before saying:

'Just notice that,'

and then start the BLS.

Interweaves using guidance from spiritual resources

During the preparation stage, make sure that you have a good idea of the client's understanding of their spiritual beliefs and resources before introducing as an interweave and only use spiritual resources that you know to be positive and will assist with their healing. Be very cautious about introducing these if your client has experienced spiritual abuse, making sure that anything you suggest is appropriate and will not retraumatise them.

Ask your client to connect in their heart before using any of the following examples:

'What do you think God would say to you?'

'Can you imagine the protection of Archangel Michael (or ask them to connect with other archangels or deities that have meaning for your client) surrounding you now?'

'Can you connect in your heart and/or soul and imagine surrendering this burden/trauma/situation/worry to the Divine?'

If you are aware that the client believes in a God that is all-loving, compassionate and non-judgemental, then you could introduce this if the client is stuck:

Client: *'God will think I am bad and deserve to be punished'* or

'I am bad or shameful in the eyes of God.'

Therapist: *'I am a bit confused; I thought I understood that God is all loving, forgiving, non-judgemental and is guiding and supporting you?'* or

'Isn't God all loving, forgiving and compassionate?' or

'What would your church or faith leader say to you about God?' or

'Connect to your heart which is the source of your inner truth. Is the God you worship forgiving, all loving, gentle and supportive?'

Of course, please change the word God to the appropriate belief that resonates with your client e.g., Divine, Buddha, Mohammed, Allah, etc.

Culturally appropriate interweaves

It may be useful to use movement as an interweave, asking your client to stretch, move part of their body or shake their body to clear some energies. Your client may find it helpful to recite a mantra, prayer, song, chant or perform another positive spiritually significant ritual that has meaning for them as part of their processing. They may like to look at an image of a positive spiritual figure, deity or a place of worship such as a temple. Remember that the aim of any interweave isn't to take the client away from the processing, but to facilitate them in continuing to stay on track with a positive resource that can support them whilst processing their distress.

Some cultures or individuals believe that it is bad to think wrong of the dead, even if they have caused significant harm. They may believe that their ancestors will hear them and inflict a spell on them or their family (Mbazzi et al., 2021). Therefore, being creative and finding suitable interweaves that take into account these beliefs is important if the processing is getting stuck or looping. It may help to invite your client to connect to their heart area which represents their inner truth, source of unconditional love, compassion for themselves and others and their authenticity. As they do this, you could ask whether they feel able to send unconditional love from their heart down their ancestral or intergenerational line and release any stress, trauma, wounds or negativity to all those who would benefit from this healing, unconditional love.

Finding somewhere suitable to release difficult emotions

Sometimes it can feel difficult for clients to express or release difficult emotions such as hatred or anger, even when applying more traditional interweaves such as a screen or soundproof box. It just may go against their values to express intense emotions to someone else even if it is emphasised that this is done within the imagination where no one could be hurt.

If this is the case, you could always ask your client whether there is a suitable safe place (which may be spiritual to them) that they can connect to in order to process the emotions and energy. Javid was an example of this in Chapter 9, where he connected with being in the ocean and could feel the soothing waters as he let go of the anger that he felt towards another person.

I have also used this technique for myself. I had been triggered in a healing session and suddenly starting to feel intense anger because I felt the healer was completely oblivious and not tuning in to what I was saying, responding with ideas that were so incongruent with my own beliefs for the situation with which I was seeking help. I wouldn't generally consider myself an angry person so the degree and depth of rage and sadness I suddenly felt seemed to be related to multiple past lives of soul trauma where I felt I hadn't been heard or understood. I also didn't feel that I could safely process the anger in normal ways, even though it would have been in the imagination. I was concerned that energetically doing this might impact and harm other people, like sending millions of energetic anger spears into the collective. When it was safe to do so and I had time to safely connect to these emotions, I decided in meditation to take myself to a distant galaxy where no life form existed. Once I felt I was in a safe, containing environment, I was then able to connect with and release the anger. It felt incredibly liberating and freeing.

Using this idea, you could invite your client to participate in something similar. As with any of the interweaves mentioned above, once offered, start the BLS and after a set, ask your client what they noticed. Often you will only need to use the spiritual interweave once or twice as this is sufficient to get the client reconnected with their adaptive network. Sometimes it may be necessary to offer an interweave or versions of the same theme of the interweave a few times as your client is learning to connect more at a heart and/or soul level. This is more likely when the client goes back into their egoic thinking (over-analysing or intellectualising), but perseverance can prove a very effective and healing intervention.

Float/bridge-back during processing

If the client becomes stuck and is looping during processing and you (or they) are sensing that there may be a past life block, then ask them to connect with the NC, emotion or body sensation that is causing the block, and ask them to float/bridge-back to the first time they experienced this in a past life (as described in Chapter 12). Once they have connected with a past life memory, continue the processing, allowing them to connect with either that memory or other related memories until the channel appears to have been cleared, that is; they are feeling calmer or connecting with positive, adaptive material for at least two BLS sets. When you bring them back to the target memory, ask them to connect to the <u>original</u> target incident and continue BLS. This should have helped clear the block and enable the processing to continue. Remember that your point of reference is the original, current target memory (and not the past life which will have been acting as a feeder memory) which will be your guide to whether processing is moving to completion.

Case example: Paul, spiritual interweave and intergenerational healing

Paul was a man in his early 30s who reported having always struggled with stress, anxiety and anger issues. He described his relationship with his mother when he was a child as caring and nurturing and his relationship with his father as good until his parents divorced when he was 11 years old. Following his parents' separation, his mother became an alcoholic and his father had a nervous breakdown, with continued mental health issues. Paul's younger brother struggled significantly with social anxiety. Paul described a tough upbringing, 'horrible,' with no money or resources, and having dyslexia meant that he struggled academically. He stopped attending school when he was around 13 years old and said he was always in trouble. When his mother was threatened with court action for his non-attendance, Paul attended a separate unit at school where they tried to support him with learning. Paul reported that his mother was out partying and taking a lot of drugs, which left him to look after his younger brother. He started work at 15 years old to get money for food as his mother spent what she had on drugs and alcohol. He managed to achieve three GCSEs and worked for a landscape gardener for five years which he enjoyed. He had been working shifts in a factory for ten years before being referred to me through his employer's insurance scheme. Paul was hardworking, committed to his job and a people pleaser, always putting others before himself. He met a woman online who lived abroad and when they plan-ned to meet up in person, the COVID-19 pandemic struck and they were unable to see each other for one and a half years, which proved a very difficult time for him. When she was able to travel, they married but it was not a happy rela-tionship, and at the time of referral, he was considering divorce. Paul also spoke about taking some psychedelics and drugs from the age of 13; he was still taking cannabis regularly and when we started working together, he was drinking every day.

Paul was rather nervous about engaging in sessions to begin with. He was struggling with work, suffering poor sleep, having angry outbursts at work because they were under-resourced, unhappy in his marriage and his beloved dog was very old and ill. Paul's main goals were to stop over-thinking, to feel calmer and less anxious. We also discussed the possibility of medication if required and I supported a referral to a psychiatrist although this proved fairly uneventful and unhelpful.

Paul watched the online workshops covering psycho-education, mind-fulness and heart led living and we went through these over a few sessions, helping him to integrate the resources into his everyday life and build up his window of tolerance. On our eighth session, I used the Feeling State Addiction protocol (Miller, 2011) to help with his dependency on alcohol which worked positively. We were then able to move towards processing some of his early memories as well as current issues around the fear of his dog dying.

The memory illustrated below was of when he was 11 years old and walked in on his mother having sex with a stranger. We worked on this memory over three separate EMDR sessions. It was the hardest trauma that he could recall in his life because it represented his mother being unavailable to him in any way (emotionally, cognitively, physically and spiritually). This had profound implications for him and his brother growing up and appeared to be a significant factor in his ongoing anger and relationship issues with others. The SUDS were reducing at the end of the second EMDR session and Paul reported being less angry with his mother and other people. His sleep was improving and he was drinking less. However, he didn't feel he would be able to release the anger to his mother as he felt what happened was inherently wrong and would always frustrate and disgust him. His frustration and hurt was specifically related to the contrast with how close he had been to his mother as a small boy and how angry and abandoned he felt when she took drugs. When we spoke about this again a few sessions later, Paul acknowledged that this memory was still triggering and impacting him, especially in relation to feelings of anger. We reviewed HLP and energies, discussing how anger is considered a much lower vibrating emotion which can make life and relationships difficult. Learning to become more heart led and authentic, which Paul was already beginning to embrace, would allow his energetic vibration to shift into a more positive place and have the possibility of healing even the deepest of wounds. Paul was keen to try some further processing of this memory, which is illustrated below, where he was able to implement and integrate HLP. In this third processing session, Paul's NC of 'I am unlovable' had changed from the initial session to 'I am not strong enough,' and his emotions had changed from anger to sadness.

Memory: Finding his mother having sex with a stranger.
Image: Seeing his brother cry.
NC: I am not strong enough.
PC: I am strong.
VOC: 2/7.
Emotions: Sad.
SUDS: 5/10.
Body location: Chest.

Below is the feedback that Paul provided after BLS sets. Any interweaves I used are shown after the word 'therapist.'

- *A lot calmer. Brother was upset. So angry with mother. She was a mess, on drugs. No matter how strong I was there is nothing I could have done.*
- *Sadness for mother. Not so much for brother as he was a baby.*
- *Calm, silence. Sorry for my mother. Then happy that she stopped as she could have caused more damage.*
- *Calm. I forgive her. I've never managed to do this before.*
- *Same. I love my mum.*

I asked Paul to reconnect with the original moment and obtained his SUDS which he reported as being 0/10. Intuitively, whilst his SUDS were 0/10, I felt his inner child was still holding on to some emotions, so I asked:

Therapist: What does your inner child feel?

- *Scared.*

Therapist: Imagine you as your Wise Self nurturing your inner child.

- *My brother is going to grandma's. I actually wish my Wise Self had been there as he would have calmed us both down.*

Therapist: Can you connect with the infinite love and support from the Divine?

- *Feeling strong. I am imagining connecting with everyone then and now with light, including my dog. It feels very positive.*
- *Calm. Inner child feels protected. No anxiety. I am there with them.*

We then moved on to the installation phase.

PC I am strong.
VOC: 5/7.

- *Calming.*
- *Grounded. VOC 7/7.*

   In the body scan he noticed positive, calming light which we strengthened with a set of BLS.

   A review at the following session confirmed the SUDS remained at 0/10. He reported having spoken to his mother about this memory which was very heal-ing for him and deepened their current relationship. His own healing, and being able to forgive his mother and release the anger, had also had a positive ener-getic impact on his mother too, suggesting some inter-generational healing. He was getting a divorce and planning to move back in with his mother to tide him over financially until he was in a better position to find a place of his own.

Case example: Daniel, spontaneously connecting with deities and soul purpose during processing

Daniel was a man in his 50s who worked in the mental health profession. He was also a mindfulness teacher working with marginalised populations. Daniel was very committed to his inner healing work and recognised that when he was in meditation for long periods of time, he re-experienced trauma symptoms from past events. He was keen to explore EMDR to help process these traumas with a therapist who also worked spiritually.

   Daniel grew up in a community that experienced high levels of social depri-vation and violence and there was violence within the family home. He was brought up within a strong Catholic community. It was a mostly positive experience but at times he found the church highly traditional, limiting and confusing. Daniel had worked in mental health services from the age of 17, including various acute mental health wards and he described losing his faith during his mental health training. He went travelling in his 20s and became interested in mindfulness and Buddhism and began to incorporate these in to his career, choosing to work with public sector staff groups and service users. Various traumas relating to his early experiences with his family, religion and early stages of career remained unprocessed, despite his spiritual and mindful practices and these traumas would be triggered during various spiritual retreats, including having flashbacks. Daniel was an incredibly sensitive and caring individual but recognised that he was carrying around a lot of shame in his energy field. When he engaged in online sessions, he reported some degree of burnout following the first year of the pandemic. When I asked about his spiritual beliefs, he said he always had a sense of Grace, a relationship with

God, Jesus, the Madonna and in adult life with Buddhism. He had been searching for meaning since a young adult. He believed he was able to link to limitless universal sources of energy at times and able to get a lot of energy from healing practices. He reported feeling very blessed.

As part of our formulation, we discussed how he may have absorbed other people's energies, not only in his community and home growing up, but also during his work in various acute and long-term mental health service settings. His peaceful place was on a ridge in the Himalayas looking out into the distance. As he connected to this place, we installed this with slow short sets of BLS and his feedback between each BLS set is illustrated below.

- *Good. Space in abdomen, warmth in chest and sense of lightness.*
- *Grounded.*
- *Solidity, ease and fearlessness. 'We are not afraid.' Vibrations in my lips which are light and gentle.*
- *'Himalaya' (the term Daniel chose to call his peaceful place).*
- *Image is very strong. Strong wind. Ease in body and sense of being connected with the elements and nature.*

The first memory we processed was in relation to the death of an inpatient when he was working on a psychiatric ward in his early 20s, and we processed this over three sessions. There was a huge sense of shame and moral confusion over what had happened on that occasion, including the failings of the service providers, but also feeling personally responsible for the death. Daniel was able to release and process this with compassion and spontaneously connect to spiritual resources, including Shiva, which enabled his heart to open and feel a great deal love. I used some Light Language at various stages during processing.

The other main incident that Daniel wanted to process was related to a situation in his 40s where he had been supporting an individual who then later refused to work with him. Three years later, this same individual had gone on to commit a murder and Daniel heard about this on television. The SUDS were not very high (possibly because of the previous sessions of EMDR) and he processed quickly, but I am illustrating this as a lovely example of how he spontaneously connected to his spiritual resources during processing to support his healing.

Memory: Friend calling me up and saying, 'look on TV.'
Image: Seeing man on TV.
NC: I am tainted.
PC: I have a heart full of compassion and care.
VOC: 2/7.
Emotions: Disgust.
SUDS: 3–4/10.
Body location: Stomach

Below is the feedback that Daniel provided after BLS sets.

- *Another image inside the flat of the man who committed the brutal murder.*
- *Disgust and aversion. Standing in the room where the murder occurred in the presence of a Buddhist monk, he shook his head and started to cry. I could feel emotions rise in me.*
- *(Tears, long set) Back in the room with the Monk – Tibetan Buddhist wheel of Life. Monk was saying 'these happenings are beyond the hell realms.' Kṣitigarbha, a Bodhisattva known as Jizo in Japanese Buddhism, who comforts beings lost in the hell realms. Crying with the monk for the terrible things that are happening in the world. 'This is your work.'*
- *(Tears, Light Language). Some nuns appeared. 'We've got this, we've got you.' Quan Yin (the female Bodhisattva of compassion). Images of birds, animals and plants.*
- *Imagining this man – no light emerging. The murder came to mind and then images of compassionate interventions that I had been a part of in other mental health settings.*

Whilst I suspected that we were close to completing the session, I closed it down as incomplete due to time constraints. We installed the most positive aspect from the processing with a few short sets of BLS:

- *It's OK to allow what is.*
- *I am further learning to understand my soul purpose.*

At the following session, we re-evaluated the SUDS which were now 0/10, so we moved to the installation phase. Daniel's PC was 'I have a heart full of compassion & care' and VOC was 7/7. We used a few sets of BLS to strengthen this:

- *Tender & buoyant energy & strength.*
- *Mind wandering. I am worthy of receiving healing & love.*
- *Buoyancy.*
- *Ease.*

In the body scan he notice energy and warmth in his face, eyes & chest. Again, a further set of BLS was applied:

- *Energy in face & body.*

Overall, the EMDR sessions had completely freed Daniel from being triggered by his past traumas and stopped the nightmares and flashbacks.

Summary

- The more aligned you as a therapist with your own authenticity, the more you will connect spiritually with your client and notice the intuitive messages that you receive during all stages of EMDR therapy, especially during the desensitisation phase.
- When appropriate and clinically justified, spiritually informed interweaves can assist clients to connect with their heart and soul and find a deeper meaning to help process their traumas.
- Clients can learn to release energies during processing that do not belong to them or that are no longer for their highest good.
- Ancestral and inter-generational healing can be achieved when clients connect in their heart and send healing energy to those generations before and after them.
- Clients can also heal past live traumas by sending healing heart energy to the different incarnations where the traumas have occurred.
- It is important to make sure that any interweave used is culturally appropriate.
- If clients appear stuck in processing and a feeder past life trauma is suspected, clients can be supported to float/bridge-back to the past life to heal the trauma and ascertain the meaning of it, so that they can integrate and learn from this in their current lifetime.

Chapter 14

EMDR Phases 5 to 8

Installation to completion

'Our faith can move mountains.'

Matthew, 17:20

This chapter covers the remaining phases of EMDR therapy including the installation, body scan, closure and re-evaluation phases. Various spiritually informed affirmations or positive statements are provided that can be used to install either as part of the Positive Cognition (PC) or at the end of an incomplete session.

Phase 5: Installation

When the SUDS (Subjective Units of Distress) have either reached 0/10 or are at an ecologically valid place, then we move on to the installation phase. For many cultures, achieving a score of 0 or 1 may seem unachievable due to the amount of trauma experienced, so please take this into account, adopting a flexible and appropriate approach. I believe that the installation phase of EMDR is one of the most important stages, because it is where we assist clients in installing a positive or preferred belief that they can start integrating into their lives, offering hope and potential for the future. From an HLP perspective, this is where significant positive change can happen *if* the client is able to integrate the learning and make heart led rather than ego led choices.

During this phase, the client is asked to connect with the original target memory or incident and check whether the PC is still valid or whether this has changed following processing. The PC may have become more spiritually meaningful or relate to areas explored in HLP, including past lives, life lessons and gifts. Examples include:

- I have a heart full of love and divine light.
- I am worthy of universal love and support.
- I have all the divine support and protection I need.
- I am divinely protected.
- I am lovingly protected and supported on my journey through life.

DOI: 10.4324/9781003509646-17

- I am learning to understand myself better.
- I am learning to heal myself.
- I am learning to live a heart led and authentic life.
- I have the strength within.
- I have everything I need within.
- I am learning to feel more integrated and whole.
- I am learning to trust the process/ my spiritual journey.
- I trust in my heart and/or soul.
- I surrender and trust in my journey.
- I trust in my highest good.
- I am open to connecting with my soul/universe/higher self/guides.
- I am embracing of my soul's journey.
- I am learning to understand my soul's purpose and mission.
- I am learning to connect with, respect, listen to or acknowledge my heart.
- I am learning to be guided by my heart.
- I am learning to find my inner truth.
- I am open to receiving love into my life.

If there was a connection with their life lesson during the course of therapy or processing sessions, then this can be part of the positive affirmation, for example:

- I am learning to have faith/trust/forgiveness/self-compassion/self-love/ acceptance, etc.
- I am open to experiencing faith/trust/forgiveness/self-compassion, etc.

Once a suitable PC is identified, the VOC is obtained. The client is asked to connect their PC with the original target memory and BLS is then applied to strengthen the VOC until it reaches 7/7. If it was already 7/7, then BLS can still strengthen this belief. If the VOC stays below 7/7, then the client is asked what prevents the PC from being completely true. I find that adding the words 'I am learning to believe' or 'I am open to the possibility of' enables the score to become more meaningful and achievable.

It may be that another memory, belief, emotion (whether from current or past life) is blocking the PC from reaching 7/7. If this is the case, this can be explored and processed, returning back to this original memory afterwards to continue with the installation and body scan (BS) phases. In some situations, clients may give a VOC score just under 7/7, either because they don't believe in extremes or they may feel they need to first perform an action to check that it is completely true. In either of these scenarios, it is appropriate to move on to the BS phase.

Clients can often have quite spiritual experiences during the installation phase as their neural network continues to make adaptive links. They may connect with spiritual resources or report experiencing spiritual feelings, images, sensations, beliefs that continue to enhance their processing.

Remember that you are the navigator, so just keep out of the way and trust in the process rather than ask too many questions at this stage that might interfere with their experiences. You can always have a short debrief at the end. As my esteemed colleague, Sandi Richman, always teaches on her EMDR trainings, 'cash in' when the client is reporting something positive to strengthen their experience.

Case example: Virág and unprocessed material emerging in the installation phase

I discussed Virág earlier in Chapter 4 where she was able to move between her heart and ego to find her truth. She was increasingly worried about her age because of a strong desire to be in a meaningly relationship and have children. Virág was spiritually and energetically aware, embracing her journey and enga- ging in regular self-care and resources. One of her blocks was finding her strength to speak her truth as this had not been encouraged as a child. We had finished processing a memory of when she was nine years old where she was trying to explain something to her mother that she disagreed with. During this EMDR ses- sion, Virág was able to forgive herself and her parents and send ancestral healing and love from her heart down the generations. This included connecting with her deceased paternal grandmother (who had a reputation of having an 'ice heart') when the energies got stuck. Virág felt she was able to heal her paternal grand- mother's blocks where she identified an inter-generational belief of not being a good parent. The processing also involved connecting to other deceased family members and social network, as well as universal support, to clear this belief and was very powerful to witness as a therapist. Although I sensed that the processing was finished, due to time constraints the session was closed as incomplete.

When we connected at the next session, I checked the SUDS and they were 0/ 10. Her PC remained the same as at the assessment stage which was 'I am as I am and can express myself freely' with a VOC of 5–6/7. Below is the feedback that Virág provided after BLS sets and any interweaves I used are shown after the word 'therapist,' illustrating that occasionally further material can arise at this stage.

- *I am back in the room. I can see my father but nothing is happening. I feel comfortable.*
- *I am quite calm. VOC: 5–6/7.*
- *I am standing there and feel stuck.*

Therapist: What needs to happen to make the words 'I am as I am and can express myself freely' (PC) feel truer?

- *I believe I need some extra validation for me to believe it. I have a small thought about whether I can trust this external opinion and won't be shut down.*

Therapist: Imagine you as your Wise Self going to be with your younger self. What would your Wise Self say to her?

- *I would say that what I am feeling is 'express yourself in a calm way. Do not let the other person's reaction influence your state of mind of being calm.' It's hard to do with the words.*
- *My mother is now talking to me because she used to shut me down and tell me not to talk, saying 'your father drank so it doesn't matter what I try.' My father is under the influence of alcohol, so it doesn't matter what I try, therefore I am blocking expressing myself.*
- *I feel like going away is not the solution so I disagree with my mother. I am not sure how to do it better.*

Therapist: Do you need other people's validation to express yourself?

- *Sometimes yes and sometimes no.*

Therapist: Do you think this is an opportunity for you to learn how to self-validate?

- *I don't always self-validate.*

Therapist: Remember it's a journey.

- *I have a tendency of falling back into things being my fault and blaming myself.*
- *Mistakes were a bad thing and caused so much trouble.*
- *I am telling my younger self to do the best she can and sit and listen to her heart and don't take it personally. That's very key. I really feel it.*
- *Strange. I have a pressure in my stomach like a little ball.*
- *I want to let it go, but don't know how.*
- *It's grey/brown in colour, the size of a tennis ball, furry with some weeds.*

(Light Language).

- *I have some light in my head. This ball only feels very small now.*
- *I feel very light, like my body is floating. The ball has gone. I am some-where in the clouds. It feels nice as if my body has lifted from the ground and is really bright.*

I checked Virág wasn't dissociating which she didn't feel the case.

- *I have an image of floating in the clouds with my body.*
- *I can be myself. VOC: 7/7.*

We then moved on to the BS where Virág reported feeling full of light and we applied some BLS to enhance this. At the following session, I re-evaluated the memory again and the SUDS remained at a 0/10, PC was 7/7, and she was overall feeling a lot better in herself from the EMDR.

Phase 6: Body Scan

This is the phase to check whether any unprocessed material is still being held within the client's body at a somatic level. This could include any stuck energies that are still being held in the client's energy field that may not necessarily belong to them, but may have been absorbed during their life. The client is asked to connect their installed PC with the original memory and mentally run a scan over their entire body and report anything they notice. If the client reports any discomfort, then BLS is applied until the discomfort subsides and reports either neutral or positive sensations. Clients may feel a desire to be more active during this phase, moving around to shake the energy out of their system. If the client reports positive sensations during the body scan, then again 'cash in' with a few short sets of BLS which may strengthen these sensations. As with the installation of the PC, clients can report a variety of responses including physical, images, positive beliefs and/or emotions, a spontaneous connection with spiritual support team or resources, spiritual symbols, etc.

Phase 7: Closure

Complete sessions

A session is considered 'complete' when the desensitisation, installation and body scan phases have been achieved. It is important to allow enough time for a debrief at the end, letting the client know that the processing may continue beyond the session. If a client connected to past lives, then a useful question to ask which may facilitate integration is:

'What has been the most important or significant lesson to take away from connecting with this past life that you can integrate into this current life?'

Make sure that it is a positive affirmation or statement, rather than something based on the trauma of what happened, in other words, you would not want to install 'I was killed for speaking out.' Examples may include:

- I can learn to speak my truth.
- I am safe now to speak my truth.
- I can be lovingly empowered to live my truth.
- I am learning to live my soul purpose.
- I am learning to understand my life lesson.
- I am learning to integrate my life lesson.
- I am learning to trust my authentic self.
- I am safe now to be my true authentic self.

Processing beyond the session may include shifts in the client's spiritual perception or changes in their energy field which may impact on relationships and situations (including work, school, activities or groups) in which they currently find themselves. As clients are healing and energetically shifting into a more positive frequency/vibration, this could impact those individuals close to them. Supporting your client to understand how this may occur is important for them so they can manage changes and keep integrating their learning. Changes could take the form of purging (physically, emotionally, spiritually and cognitively) which is not an uncommon experience on a spiritual journey as part of the ongoing healing process. Purging is an opportunity to eliminate what is no longer needed for the client's highest good; are they able to utilise what they are beginning to learn from their heart and authenticity or does their ego tempt them to re-engage with old habits and beliefs? Encourage your client to use their resources and practise healthy self-care in all areas of their life including diet, exercise, mindfulness, etc. They may have opportunities between sessions to practise their life lesson/s including setting out clearer boundaries or being empowered to speak their truth or experience having more self-worth.

Make sure that your client leaves the session in a stable, safe and grounded place. You could use any of the previous exercises or strategies mentioned throughout this book.

Incomplete sessions

It is not unusual for EMDR processing to be incomplete at the end of a session, depending on complexity of trauma and time available. However, I always encourage supervisees to let go of any expectations or assumptions of how they think the session may progress, because some clients can process very fast and intensely. I have noticed that clients who are more spiritually aware and implementing regular self-care into their lives can process quickly, as well as when there is a strong spiritual resonance created between therapist and client.

It is essential to always leave sufficient time to conclude the session with the intention that the client will depart feeling as calm and contained as possible and in a much stronger place than they arrived. I never check SUDS at the end of the session if I haven't enough time to finish any further processing that may be required or to complete the installation and BS stages. Therapists who do check SUDS at the end of sessions are generally curious about how well the processing has gone, but this will be coming from their ego and can pose a dilemma. What happens if the client still rates the SUDS highly? Both the client and therapist may feel that something has gone wrong or that the client isn't making progress. It may sound obvious, but SUDS are subjective; a 1 or 2/10 could take another one or two sessions to process depending on the meaning for the client of what that number represents. I am therefore encouraging you not to try and rush the process but to trust and surrender to divine timings. I have had many clients where I suspect we are near the end of the processing but have little time left for closure. I will therefore make the choice to finish the BLS at a place where the client is in a neutral or calm place and then close the session down as incomplete. At the following appointment, I ask the client to reconnect with the original memory and repeat the assessment stage, as the client's responses may have changed between sessions. I then continue with processing until complete. Sometimes, when a session has been closed as incomplete due to time constraints, even though I intuitively felt the trauma has been completely processed, when we re-assess the memory at the following session, the SUDS are 0/10. We are then in a position and have more time to move on move into the installation and body scan phases.

Something I have found incredibly beneficial and that I use routinely is to ask the client:

'What has been the most helpful or important thing that you can take away from today's processing?'

We are not searching for a positive statement or affirmation that is the same as their original PC although sometimes this can happen. We are attempting to ascertain how the processing has given some insight into how the client views their experiences and what the positive meaning is for them. The client may give some feedback about what the processing experience was like for them or a particular moment that felt quite pertinent. They may also say something about how hard or emotional it has been and if this is the case, I would look at rephrasing this to a positive statement, asking the client:

'Knowing that you have started to process and connect with this, what does that make you believe about yourself?'

This question facilitates the client to connect with something positive but they may need further assistance so I might offer a few suggestions such as:
'I am wondering if that makes you realise or believe that:

- *I am learning to connect and work through this, or*
- *I am strong enough to release the distress,*
- *I can begin to believe I will get through this,*
- *I am starting to embrace my healing journey.'*

There are a whole host of positive affirmations that one can use (see the examples provided earlier in this chapter).

Once you have established a positive phrase or statement, then install it with a short, slow set of BLS. Clients usually report that this is a very positive experience and are ready to leave the session in a lighter mood.

Other options for closing down the session could include using familiar previously installed resources, for example, safe/peaceful place, container, connection with spiritual resource team, etc. You may decide to finish the session with a prayer, mantra, mudra, oracle card reading, sound healing or other forms of energy work. I have used Light Language for some clients where I intuitively feel some of this energy coming through and that can be a powerful way to close down sessions energetically.

Whether the session is complete or incomplete, clients are asked to keep a record or journal of any unprocessed material or memories that may surface between sessions. From a spiritual perspective, clients are encouraged to notice and journal any changes, including energetic, within themselves. I encourage clients to utilise the elements of HLP, taking the role of the observer as to whether they are having opportunities to practise life lessons, the choices they make, and the impact these have on their relationships and situations.

Spiritual support team stopping the processing

It is also important to be aware that whilst the client may have given verbal agreement for soul level work, very occasionally the client's ego could be making the choice rather than their heart and soul. Egos can be tricksters at times! It is unusual but it may happen. It may not be in the best interest for the client's soul to participate in specific soul level healing at certain times, so if the session doesn't quite go as anticipated, trust the process and divine timings.

Case example: Bella and an incomplete session where her soul or spiritual support stopped the processing

This is the only session where I felt a client's soul, guide or support team actively intervened to stop the processing. I was working with a client, Bella, on some of her traumas involving attachment difficulties with parents, previous abusive relationships and OCD behaviours. Bella had grown up not being allowed to express her emotions, so had spent her life being highly dissociated from them. She was a spiritually insightful person, very focused on her soul purpose and journey. Bella had engaged well with HLP, resource work and was becoming more mindful and present in everyday life. Sessions were undertaken online and she used the butterfly taps for BLS. We had completed seven sessions very successfully before Bella felt ready to process the death of one of her children who had been stillborn 11 years previously. During this session, Bella was finding it hard to connect with the memory which was unusual for her. After several BLS sets, I asked what was good about not connecting with the memory to which she replied, 'not having to deal with how I felt.' I shortened the length of BLS sets using the CIPOS approach so that we could just dip in to the memory for ten seconds at a time to see if that made it more manageable to connect. This helped her to connect to a memory of what had been happening in the abusive relationship with the child's father before experiencing the stillbirth. After the next BLS, Bella said:

- *I can feel someone touching my face (in the session). It doesn't feel negative, but it's the second time it has happened in this session.*

We continued with the processing, still having shorter sets, with Bella connecting to different memories in connecting to the child's father before the stillbirth. After a few more sets Bella said:

- *I can feel someone pulling my hand. It feels like someone is trying to stop me connecting with it.*
- *Feels as if someone is saying 'not now.'*

We agreed to stop the processing and had a debrief. I emphasised to Bella that it was important we acknowledged what was happening in a positive way. Maybe one of her guides or her soul was just saying that today was not the right time and it was important for us to respect this without trying to over-analyse it. We reflected on how previous EMDR processing sessions had been very smooth and successful so what she had just experienced was not a typical occurrence. The most important thing that Bella could take away from this session was 'what is meant for me won't pass me and I trust my own instincts' which we installed at the end of the session.

We had an EMDR session the following week and she agreed to re-connect with this memory again. It ended up being a powerful session with lots of processing. Bella was able to experience the raw emotions and start the healing from this trauma, connecting with her Wise Self to assist in the processing. The session was incomplete but the most important thing that Bella could take away was 'I am learning to safely connect to my emotions' which we installed at the end of the session. At the next session, Bella reported the SUDS from the memory of her daughter's death were 0/10. Her PC was 'I am strong' which we installed and had a VOC of 7/7. In her body scan, Bella reported feeling a comforting, tight hug around her arms, which we installed.

This is Bella's version of events that happened that day:

'I remember attending one of my EMDR sessions with the intention to cover a topic I had feared but knew it was time to work through. However, as the process started, every time I tried to recover the experience in my mind/memory, I felt a hand on my shoulder. It was neither intimidating nor frightening, but it did seem to block the vision I was trying to work through. I tried several times to work past it, but this warm, calming pressured hand would do the same thing. I realised, along with Alexandra, that this was not the time. I was not ready, and something, someone, was kindly allowing me not force anything I was not ready for. Alexandra and I spoke about the experience, and we agreed,

for now, that we would reserve this particular traumatic experience, and revisit. The following week, I managed to work through that same traumatic experience. There were no hands upon my shoulder, but clear visual representations of my past. I was able to process clearly and successfully.'

Perhaps this case shows how important it is to trust and surrender to the process, the client's soul and divine timings and not to become too attached or over-analyse these experiences. Healing will occur at the right time.

Phase 8: Re-evaluation

At the next session it is important to check in with your client and see what may have arisen between sessions. They may have recorded or journalled new memories or material that they would like to work on. They may have experienced various changes (e.g., emotional, spiritual, cognitive or physical) during their week that they would benefit from sharing with you. It is also important to re-evaluate the memory you previously worked on. Even if it had finished as a complete session, I re-check the SUDS to determine whether any material has re-surfaced that still needs processing. If the session was closed as incomplete, I ask the client to re-connect with the target memory, go through the assessment questions (as these areas may have changed since we last worked on the memory) and continue with processing until completion.

Repair

Being a therapist is not an exact science. We are human beings first and foremost and it is not about getting it right or conducting a perfect EMDR session because that just isn't realistic or achievable, certainly not all of the time. The spiritual journey is about embracing opportunities to learn, grow, develop and explore new creative ways to advance your practice, whilst also staying true to the fundamental tenets of EMDR. Mistakes will happen, whether it is because you are new to EMDR or perhaps because you are going through your own challenges at the time. Learning to accept yourself and know that you are doing the best you can at any given stage with the tools, resources and support available to you is essential. Owning mistakes, staying humble in your approach and being prepared to heal your inner wounds is also vital to progress into a more authentic, heart led approach in all areas of your life. Clients will be your mirrors and teachers to you, some stronger than others. If mistakes are made but you have established a safe, containing, therapeutic relationship then create space within sessions to repair those mistakes with your client. Repair can be very healing and you will also be acting as a role model for your client. Occasionally you will have clients who may have highly complex personalities or be so dissociative or unable to work through this so whatever you say or do will never be enough. If this is the case, you still have the option of sending love from your heart to theirs or perhaps you can use the Hawaiian prayer keeping them in mind. Establish healthy boundaries, make sure you have effective support, regular supervision and maintain clear records of your therapeutic work.

Summary

- The installation phase enables a positive or preferred belief to be strengthened when connected to the original target memory and this can be of spiritual significance for the client.
- Clients can have spiritual experiences during the installation and body scan, including connecting with deities, spiritual resource team, healing lights and heightened, positive body sensations.
- It is beneficial to install a positive meaningful statement or affirmation at the end of incomplete sessions which may be spiritually based.
- Trust in divine timings and that clients will process and heal at the right time on their spiritual journey.
- Be open to repair when you make mistakes and remain humble in your approach.

Chapter 15

Other considerations in EMDR therapy

'Set your life on fire. Seek those who fan your flames.'

Rumi

The aim of this final chapter is to cover some additional areas about working spiritually with EMDR clients. Firstly, the three-pronged approach within the EMDR framework is discussed with an emphasis on the importance of integrating the healing and learning from EMDR trauma therapy. How to introduce HLP ideas into EMDR supervision is then covered. A summary of the main considerations to take into account when working within a cultural framework with any client is then provided. I conclude with highlighting a few additional topics where I have a little bit more experience or knowledge including adopting a spiritual and energetical approach when working online, with children, within neurodiversity and the use of psychedelics, illustrated with case studies. There are of course many areas that could be deemed relevant but where I lack clinical or personal experience, space is left for other therapists to fill those gaps, sharing ideas, knowledge and wisdom for the future. I hope that this is an area that can grow, expand and be as inclusive as possible.

Three-pronged protocol

Taking a three-pronged approach to our EMDR therapy is part of standard accredited EMDR training as discussed by Shapiro (2018). It addresses past, current and future traumas within one's case conceptualisation and treatment plan. In an ideal situation, one would first address unprocessed traumas from the past which are still impacting on current distress. The current situations or triggers that are activating the present distress are then targeted. Once this has been completed and if clients are still reporting current anxiety, then 'flashforwards' (Logie & De Jongh, 2014) is a useful technique to employ. This is where clients are asked to imagine the worst possible scenario in the future to a presently held fear. Some clients, often deeply anxious ones, will have created a script or narrative in their

DOI: 10.4324/9781003509646-18

'thought bubbles' of an imagined scenario in the future which continues to impact on them. I had a client who feared meeting a perpetrator in the afterlife, so we connected with her imagined scenario using the flashforwards procedure and processed this with great success.

Finally, the positive future template, or protocol, can be used to facilitate a healthy adaptive response to future tasks. Using the positive future template, clients can connect with the various spiritual resources available to them to find mastery when imagining dealing with future challenges, situations or when making new, heart led authentic choices. For complex clients, it is important to have flexibility in what to target first so they can build up trust and resilience in using EMDR. Severe trauma and attachment difficulties from an early age can impair cerebral development, making it much harder for these individuals to achieve optimal neurological and mental functioning. Gonzalez & Mosquera (2012) described adopting a progressive approach to EMDR therapy when working with severely dissociative clients.

The three-pronged approach applies when working spiritually with our clients but can also be extended beyond this current life timeline, connecting with past lives, ancestral or inter-generational traumas and healing them at a soul and energetic level. Integrating the learning and gifts is an essential component of HLP and one's spiritual journey, leading to the adoption of new heart led choices rather than retreating into old, familiar patterns. In other words, making the unfamiliar, familiar. The opportunities to practise this from a spiritual perspective will continue far beyond the processing of past or current blocks or traumas. It is highly likely that clients will find themselves in situations where they are given 'tests' to see whether they are able to put their learning into practice. At times this can be challenging as old NCs are triggered. Previous repetitive themes or scenarios may resurface, rather like peeling away the layers of an onion, to give clients the chance to make different choices that are more in alignment with their heart and authenticity. Learning to become an observer, to step out of the scenario and apply HLP is crucial when creating alternative, more positive outcomes. Therefore, clients may benefit from further support where the therapist takes on the role of spiritual coach or mentor. Navigating the spiritual journey can be tough, especially if someone is very determined to be more authentic in their life. It is essential that clients learn to maintain daily self-care strategies to work through the changes that happen to them in their relationships and situations in life rather than spiritually bypass. This may include making significant changes in such as leaving a job, relationships or making changes to friendships or activities that are no longer energetically in alignment with their heart. Sometimes EMDR therapy can assist with these changes by identifying any blocks or fears that may be getting in the way. With time, the client learns to have self-trust, self-confidence and manage such changes with less external support.

Case example: Billie and integration

Billie had processed many different traumas including rape. At a review session, she described feeling much happier and bubbly in herself, more resilient and she felt her energies were really high and joyous. I noticed a difference in her energetically and commented about how lovely she looked and appeared. Billie had been struggling to engage at work for several years, but in the past few weeks she had observed a positive effect when connecting with her colleagues, saying:

'The higher energy that I am bringing into work is being attracted back to me. I am getting on with people so much better and even attending outside work events which was unheard of before. People are commenting about how different I seem. When I look back at my text messages to my sister last year, they were full of comments about how much I hated working.'

Billie also shared how she was enjoying using the resources and self-care techniques as this was her commitment to herself and she commented on the joy it was bringing in to her life. I discussed with her the importance of continuing with daily self-care, taking the observer role and noticing when she might be tempted to repeat old, familiar patterns of trauma and challenge. This helped her to believe that she was able to make new choices in life moving forwards by making healthier unfamiliar experiences become the norm.

Case example: Daniel and integration

Here is an example of how the Light Language used in my sessions with Daniel (see the case detailed in Chapter 13) continued to impact on him a year after we finished. Daniel shared with me an experience he had whilst on holiday.

'Whilst I was walking in the Alps, after a long, steep climb I crossed an alpine meadow full of late spring flowers. I then dropped down into a wooded valley with a wide stream and some small waterfalls with sunlight glimmering off the water. Quite spontaneously I started to hear your voice in "the mind's ear" speaking Light Language. I tuned in and just enjoyed and appreciated it. It lasted a minute or so and then recurred a few times for a few seconds whilst I was by the stream. Shortly after I crossed a bridge over the stream. The bridge name translated to English as the bridge of faeries. Just a lovely moment.'

HLP in EMDR supervision

The principles of HLP can be applied to any situation that is challenging, including the home environment, work or organisational challenges. I also use the ideas of HLP in supervision sessions when appropriate, supporting supervisees when they are being triggered by their clients, or feeling stuck within themselves, to explore what the situation is trying to teach, learn or heal. I may encourage the supervisee to reflect what their client could be mirroring back to them and any of their unprocessed material that would be beneficial to work through outside of supervision. I have applied HLP when supervisees are struggling with organisational difficulties in order to facilitate them in understanding what they could learn from systemic challenges. Teaching supervisees to notice and differentiate the messages from their ego, heart and/or soul can help them to respect and honour their heart and/or soul, rather than feel bound by the ego's hooks and expectations. This may enable supervisees to have a healthier outlook on their work circumstances in order to make informed decisions that feel more authentic.

I also encourage supervisees to connect with their intuition to observe the energetic connection with their client and how this can provide useful information to guide them in their work. I was in peer supervision with a couple of colleagues, one of whom was interested in exploring his 'blind spot' when working with clients. He mentioned having had a supervisor 20 years previously who told him he was like a fox-terrier and while his intuitive assumptions were mostly correct, it could make him dangerous. Since that comment, my colleague had become much more cautious about listening to his inner guidance, as if he had been 'shut down and silenced.' I reflected back how sad I was to have heard his story as he was a very mindful, insightful person and that possibly his supervisor found him a threat because his supervisor was lacking in intuition. It really highlighted to me the significance of the words we convey to others in all areas of our work and lives and the importance of consciously owning and working through our own issues rather than projecting them onto others.

Cultural considerations and adaptations

I have attempted to weave various cultural adaptations that may be required into the EMDR standard protocol throughout the book. However, I also acknowledge that there will be areas that I may have missed so please explore and adapt according to the individual that you are working with. I mentioned in Chapter 2 the importance of being culturally competent which applies to all areas of our work and includes a commitment to learning to implement a non-judgemental, anti-oppressive practice and have knowledge of as wide as possible a range of lived experiences (Khan, 2023). As part of this process, using self-reflection, support through supervision, and HLP concepts, we start to recognise and manage our own bias, become aware of our blind spots, unconscious and conscious biases that might impact the energetic or spiritual relationship with our clients.

Various studies have also been published to suggest cultural adaptations to both the individual and group EMDR protocols for different continents around the world (see e.g., Jarero et al., 2014; Mehrotra, 2014). Below is a summary based on Mbazzi et al.'s (2021) research findings from the experience of EMDR therapists working within five African countries, including some of the adaptations they recommend. Many of these recommendations also apply to complex clients, irrespective of their cultural, spiritual or religious backgrounds:

- Use culturally appropriate metaphors when explaining trauma and EMDR.
- Make sure you are culturally competent to assist in building a strong, therapeutic alliance.
- Incorporate spiritual or religious practices during the session, for example, you may start with a prayer, mantra, blessing or meditation.
- Use a lifeline technique when completing the history-taking and select only a few target memories when establishing your treatment plan so as not to overwhelm clients.
- Allow resourcing to be interwoven throughout the therapeutic process to facilitate stabilisation, safety and containment, rather than just reserving this for Phase 2 of EMDR therapy.
- Be careful with how you describe the 'safe' place exercise and other resourcing exercises (e.g., container) and use appropriate terminology that resonates for your client.
- Where possible, incorporate spiritual or cultural ideas, including movement, dance, connection with a higher source (God, Divine, Allah, etc.) throughout the EMDR therapy process.
- Find a stop signal that your client is comfortable with or check in with them more regularly if they feel unable to use a stop signal.
- Use simple language and explanations, recognising that some cultures may not understand or be able to verbalise concepts such as NC, PC and emotions.
- When ascertaining scores on the rating scales, be flexible and consider using hand movements, pictures or visual options, colours, etc. as alternative methods to rate the scales. Do not expect SUDS to reach 0 or 1.
- Be flexible with the type of BLS used.
- Take care when doing the BS as this can trigger other traumatic material.
- Using spiritual interweaves can be very powerful and beneficial.
- Be aware of potential power dynamics between you and your client and the position you represent as the therapist.
- Some cultures may feel more comfortable working with someone of the same gender.
- Certain cultures may also find making eye contact difficult or struggle to show signs of emotion as this may not be encouraged or permitted.
- If possible, and with the client's permission, collaborate with indigenous healers or faith leaders who may also be providing some support and healing.

Clients may choose to work with someone from their own faith or cultural background. However, they may also intentionally choose to work with someone outside of this, especially if they are questioning their faith or beliefs or if they are concerned about being judged if they discuss their difficulties within their own community. This highlights the importance of creating a safe environment for your client to share and explore what is happening for them in an open-minded supportive way so that they can find their own truth and authenticity.

Working online

Some therapists were actively using EMDR successfully online before the global pandemic in 2020. I think it is fair to say that when global lockdowns occurred by late March of that year, most of us suddenly had to change the way we worked and learn how to adapt EMDR for online sessions. There was an initial pause in EMDR accredited trainings with concern that trainee EMDR therapists would not have a full experience of using EMDR by practising eye movement in person. We quickly had to adapt the way BLS was offered, using self-tapping methods such as the 'Butterfly Hug' (introduced by Artigas et al., 2000), or various online programmes that could deliver eye movements or auditory BLS. I did not notice a significant change in the quality of my EMDR therapy; clients managed to process in a similar way to in person sessions and it also opened up my practice to a larger group of people around the world.

There were a few challenges I faced and still have to work through. I noticed that it is not always as easy to spot the subtle nuances in a client; you usually only see part of their physical body, noticing that a small tear, a change in facial colouring or expression was less apparent. I soon realised that energetically I was having to work much harder at connecting and attuning to the client at a level that I aspired to achieve to facilitate maximum healing potential in the session. This impacted on my overall energy levels and I certainly experienced what became known as 'Zoom fatigue.' This meant that I had to adjust the timings of my sessions to allow longer breaks between clients and I had to reduce the number of clients I saw in a week. It was around this time that I increased my level of self-care each day to around two to three hours, with plenty of opportunities to ground myself and connect with the outdoors and with nature. I had to stop facilitating online EMDR trainings, as well as attending online training courses that spanned several days, because the intensity of the experience led to severe headaches and migraine. I interpreted this as my body telling me it wasn't healthy for me to spend such long periods of time at the computer.

The other significant challenge concerned the technical issues. I have always had an interesting relationship with technology and it used to be a very quick trigger that spiralled me into an emotional heap! Fundamentally, it is what the trigger represents. Not only does technology send my Attention Deficit Hyperactivity Disorder (ADHD) type brain into a scramble and overwhelm, but it is also important that the technology functions smoothly, otherwise it impacts on my work and income. When it goes wrong, I used to quickly enter my thought bubble where my ego would create wonderful stories about how I was going to lose everything, become homeless and derelict. It is quite funny when I think about it at times, but in moments when I really do need the technology to work, it can be intense and an effective trigger to my core internal wounds. I have an awareness of this now and as I keep working on myself, the trigger is much less powerful and usually operates at a level of minor annoyance as I know that I am able to fix things eventually.

Technical issues do occur however. I cannot say for definite that this happens more frequently when working spiritually with clients, but I know from discussing this with other colleagues and friends, that they have noticed similar occurrences. For example, when connecting with a client and discussing significant spiritual concepts that may be pertinent to them, the internet connection fails or the sound mysteriously stops or other such phenomena. It is as if the energy being transmitted via words or attunement results in a temporary crash in the system. I am sure you already do, but it is wise to have a backup option, using a different programme or device. I try to simply observe the synchronicities of these events, whilst also paying more attention to my work and being a little more prepared so that I can continue to function as best as possible, especially during EMDR processing sessions.

Before the pandemic, I had already experienced online healing sessions, especially Light Language, with healers across the globe, so I trusted that healing could happen energetically despite different time zones and technical factors. Below is an example of how one of my clients, Javid, who was discussed previously in Chapter 9, commented on the power of the healing during one of his online sessions.

Case example: Javid working online and introducing Light Language during processing

We were working on a memory when Javid was ten years old and had got caught up in a fight at school when I intuitively felt some Light Language come through during the processing. He was recognising how he felt he had soaked up so many emotions from others in his life. I had never spoken about Light Language before this session, and whilst it is not ideal to bring into the middle of a processing session, sometimes it comes through strongly, so I have learnt to trust the divine timings.

Memory: Ten years old in a fight at school.
Image: Friends laughing at me.
NC: I am weak.
PC: I am strong.
VOC: 1/7.
Emotions: Embarrassed, crying.
SUDS: 8/10.
Body location: Chest and throat.

During the first few sets, the image disappeared quickly and Javid was left with the emotions and physical sensations, to which we used heart interweaves (connecting to his heart) to facilitate the processing. I introduced the option of Light Language, to which Javid agreed and was very excited about. Below illustrates the feedback in between sets of BLS obtained from Javid both before and after the Light Language.

- *Thought of observing energy from others. I get negative energy from others easily, very easily, it's like a magnet drawing the negative energy from others.*

Therapist: Introduced Light Language

- *(Light Language). I have so many questions. What just happened, what was that language, and how? The only sensation I am feeling is that the pressure in my jaw, chin and mouth are disappearing completely, I feel like I am about to burst into tears and I don't know why and I don't understand a single word you said and this is all happening in real life and the other side of the screen and how? What is this, what is the logic in any of this?*

Both of us shared a lovely moment of lightness and laughter because Javid was very intellectual and logical and I had previously explained when introducing Light Language that his biggest challenge would be to stay out of his head and just allow the Light Language to flow. I said that we could debrief at the end of the session, encouraging him to keep going with the processing as it seemed to be helping to release some of the emotions.

- *(Light Language). Struggling to keep my eyes open, flame in my chest is going down. There is still a bit of pain in my jaw but as I took a deeper breath the pressure decreased.*
- *(Light Language). Energy is coming down my face, bit blocked still in my jaw. Little bit of burning in stomach although barely noticeable and just a sensation.*
- *(Light Language). I am blinking a lot. All the pressure has disappeared. Feeling very chilled and calm.*

The session was incomplete but the most positive aspect from the processing that Javid reported was 'I can be very happy' which we installed. When we reviewed this at the following session, Javid's SUDS were 0/10, so we moved to the installation phase. His PC was 'I am strong' (VOC 6/7).

- *Same belief.*
- *Same belief. (VOC 7/7).*

In the body scan he noticed a little pressure in his jaw.

- *Not there anymore. Relaxed.*

Working with children

Aspects of working spiritually with children have been discussed throughout the book and I am much more mindful about the language I use with children when exploring this topic. If you know that they like connecting with crystals, aromatherapy oils, dream catchers, nature, prayers or spiritual healing rituals, then these can be resourced during the preparation phase of EMDR. Be curious when working with children from different cultures and faiths as to positive spiritual or cultural important resources and see if there are opportunities to introduce these if appropriate and realistic (i.e., they are supported by their social circumstances and environment).

Client example: Providing a safe environment for children

A mother of a ten-year-old boy contacted me asking for sessions for her son who had been struggling with anxiety for several years. He had previously had a few sessions online with another therapist during the pandemic but his mother was keen for him to engage with someone in person. I suspected from her initial email that there was quite a bit of information to gather and she was unsure whether her son would engage, so I suggested meeting her first to gather all the relevant information and then we could decide if I was the right person. At our initial appointment, she told me how sensitive her son was to many things including teachers, foods, materials, etc. and whilst there were some similar traits with ASD (Autistic Spectrum Disorder), she said the GP had ruled this out following a screening procedure. There were definite indications of separation anxiety with parents, heightened because the mother had a chronic health condition. She said she had shown her son a small online video of my clinic room and he was somewhat anxious about my large Buddha painting but she felt it was worth trying to bring him to a session. When he arrived a few weeks later, I let him explore the room and examine its contents so that he could ask questions and let me know whether there were things he didn't feel comfortable with. He showed great interest in the crystal bowls so I retrieved some from the shelf and we both took turns to play them. I asked him to notice what it felt like in his body as he listened to the sound. He reported feeling calmer and he particularly resonated with the green heart chakra bowl. He loved the variety of crystals on the table and told me how he was a regular visitor to the local natural health shop and would select crystals that he was instinctively drawn too. He also pointed out the chimes in my room, so I played these and again asked what he noticed in his body, reporting back that it made him feel calm. Once settled into the space, we were then able to explore in more detail his daily worries and behaviour. I discussed with him and his mother about the possibility of exploring some sound healing, maybe by attending sound healing gong baths or purchasing some sound healing objects as part of his ongoing resources in addition to our sessions.

Neurodiversity

At the time of writing this book, the area of neurodiversity is a hot topic. More and more individuals of all ages are seeking a diagnosis to explain symptoms that they have been struggling with for many years and the number of clients looking for additional therapeutic support who consider themselves as neurodiverse has significantly increased.

It is not the aim of this book to explore in depth why there is an increase in people identifying themselves as neurodiverse and I am sure there are many explanations or theories being proposed. I do wonder about the change and speed of lifestyle which in turn creates such a demand on individuals. From an educational perspective, the old, traditional ways of teaching have insisted on fitting children into boxes, expecting them to sit still for long periods of time, perhaps in over-stimulating environments. When I was at school, many of my lessons involved being dictated to and having to somehow capture and write this information down. Not only was this exceptionally boring, but my brain really struggled to convert what I was hearing to paper. I knew I struggled but didn't realise I had the strong traits associated with dyslexia and ADHD so this created the belief that I was stupid. This will be a familiar story to many but somehow, I managed to get by and gradually learnt techniques to manage, mask or avoid certain situations.

I also hold a level of curiosity about the overlaps between symptoms of neurodiversity and people considering themselves to be energetic, spiritual or highly sensitive persons. Examples include:

- Heightened sensitivities to sounds, smells, visions, touch, emotions and textures which can feel overwhelming.
- Feeling different or not fitting in.
- Challenges with technology or information processing.
- Noticing one's energy change with certain situations or with people, creating a rush of energy or complete exhaustion.
- Heightened perception.
- Interpreting information in a different way; some individuals see people in colours, others report reading energy fields and auras.
- Needing time alone to recharge.
- Addictive behaviour.
- Difficulty being grounded.
- Tendency to absorb energies like a sponge.
- Difficulties concentrating and poor memory.
- Vivid imagination.
- Gastro-intestinal issues.
- Gynaecological issues.
- Empathic.
- Intuitive.

However, whilst there is an overlap, there are also clear differences including social interactions, communication styles and repetitive behaviour. In addition, individuals who have dual or multiple diagnoses such as ADHD and ASD tend to exhibit a mixture of traits that do not always complement each other. For example, the hyperactive part of them may make them seek out social interactions and appear bubbly, gregarious and lively, whereas the ASD part of them may prefer being on their own and engaging in more solitary behaviours.

There is no reason to believe that a neurodiverse person is any more or less spiritual than a neurotypical person. I have worked with clients and have friends and colleagues who would consider themselves both very spiritual and neurodiverse. Many of the spiritual healers that I have had sessions with would consider themselves as neurodiverse. If I was forced to put myself into a category, which I am trying to do less so in life, I would probably describe myself as a highly sensitive person.

Using EMDR with neurodiverse spiritual individuals is no different. We adopt a unique perspective and learn to attune to what life is like for them, what works and doesn't work and support them in finding the tools to manage the challenges. Mindfulness has made a considerable improvement in my quality of life, helping me to understand and manage my energy levels and enabling me to function more effectively. Adopting a heart led life is also essential to finding self-love, understanding life lessons and the gifts to embrace through different experiences. As with all spectrums, some neurodiverse individuals will readily understand and embrace spirituality and HLP, whilst with others it may not resonate at all.

I have observed that some neurodiverse clients, especially clients with ADHD, may process quite rapidly and powerfully in sessions. In addition, I have noticed that significant change, shifts and insights can occur between appointments and when they come back after an incomplete processing session, other issues or areas of their life are at the forefront which they want to talk or work through, rather than wanting to go back to previous incomplete material. Adopting a client-centred approach could easily lead to several different memories being worked on without reaching completion, so it is important to be aware this may happen and at regular intervals, review the targeted EMDR memories and explain to clients why it is beneficial to try and complete processing.

Psychedelics

The area of psychedelics is increasing in popularity and momentum, with Australia becoming the first country to legalise medical psychedelics in 2023 to treat some persistent mental health conditions. Many research trials are being conducted on the benefits of psychedelic assisted therapy especially with complex conditions such as treatment resistant depression, anorexia nervosa, addictions, PTSD, chronic pain and obsessive-compulsive disorder. This is exciting and offers hope to clients who have struggled to heal with traditional psychotherapy or medical intervention. The interest in integrating EMDR therapy with psychedelics has also grown and EMDR can provide a highly effective therapy to assist both in the preparation before taking psychedelics, as well as the integration afterwards. Various EMDR clinicians have presented and written about psychedelic assisted psychotherapy and EMDR especially since 2020 (e.g., Raine-Smith & Rose, 2025).

The reason why I am touching on this topic in this book is that psychedelics may be used by some individuals as part of their spiritual journey and can result in a range of different outcomes. Television documentaries, such as Michael Pollan's *How to Change Your Mind*, have brought the awareness of psychedelics into many households. The most popular psychedelics are psilocybin, LSD, ayahuasca/DMT, peyote, MDMA and ketamine and some individuals pay a great deal of money and travel great distances to participate in psychedelic retreats. Clients may experiment with micro-dosing. Others will experiment with psychedelics on their own or attend 'underground' events. They may be just curious about exploring what happens during psychedelic use, others may have the intention of connecting with a higher presence or different realms and some may believe that it will clear and heal deep underlying trauma without the necessity of additional therapeutic work. Therefore, it is a helpful question to routinely ask clients as part of the initial history-taking phase about any psychedelic usage during their life. Ask when they did this and ascertain what their experience was like and ascertain whether additional processing may be beneficial using EMDR as part of the treatment package you offer.

Where clients have had a positive experience during a psychedelic trip, this could represent a moment that is resourced in the preparation stages of EMDR, for example, feeling a connection with a higher presence, deities, nature or a sense of 'oneness' with their surroundings. Whilst there may be many potential benefits that clients report from using psychedelics if used carefully, and integrated within healthy self-care practices or additional therapeutic support, there is always a danger that for some it can result in spiritual crisis. I have had a few clients with complex histories of traumas and ongoing psychological difficulties who have attended psychedelic retreats abroad and were not prepared or resourced at all.

Client example: Juliana's experience of spiritual crisis after a psilocybin retreat

Juliana attended a psilocybin retreat after her then husband had seen Michael Pollan's documentary and thought it would be a good idea to help resolve her psychological issues. Juliana had been on anti-depressants for nine years. The first time I heard from her was when she contacted me three weeks after her retreat in a crisis. She was feeling suicidal, off work sick and suffering many underlying health issues. She told me that the support offered from the retreat organisers was available at £300 per session which was unaffordable and unsustainable. Fortunately, she had health insurance cover and I had space to pick her up quickly and offer some intense sessions to ground, resource and stabilise her. We were then in a position to start EMDR processing during session nine. We had over 40 sessions in total, with many of these focused on supporting Juliana through her spiritual journey using the ideas behind HLP. As Juliana grew stronger, she was in a position to take leaps of faith including moving house, leaving her marriage and starting a new relationship. Many of the EMDR sessions focused on her poor attachment relationship with her parents, especially her mother, where her underlying NCs of unworthiness and not being good enough were still impacting her everyday life. Over time, Juliana's daily self-care increased significantly and she stopped micro-dosing. We were also able to successfully process a past miscarriage using heart interweaves which she had previously tried to work through on her own using psilocybin.

Not exclusive to psychedelic retreats, as this can happen in any spiritual gathering or healing retreat, I know of spiritually aware clients who have had traumatic experiences as a result of the lack of appropriate support or attunement from some facilitators. This may result in spiritual crisis or spiritual abuse because of the breach of trust and safety during the experience, sometimes resulting in a deep questioning of a person's own spiritual understanding and fundamental meaning behind life. All of these traumas can be areas that benefit from EMDR processing.

Are there times when HLP is not appropriate?

As with any of the work we offer, it is important to reflect on the reasons why we introduce a therapy or a particular way of working with clients. I don't believe in fitting clients into boxes, but instead in finding the right approach for them that is tailored to their needs and requirements. This also applies when considering using HLP with clients. There is no harm at all in asking about a person's spiritual beliefs, so long as you, as a therapist, are respectful and open and work with your client's belief system without imposing your own views.

I believe HLP can be utilised with clients who are open-minded, motivated and have a certain level of psychological insight. However, extra care and caution needs to be taken when working with clients who have fragile, complex personalities or are highly dissociative as they may not have the cognitive strength to understand or apply aspects of HLP. If your client is actively suicidal or psychotic, then obviously stabilisation must take priority. Risk management has to take precedence, as with any other therapy or intervention offered. Once all risks have been managed appropriately and your client is more stable and able to engage in a therapeutic way, then it is probably safe to introduce HLP.

Undertaking any soul level work using soul therapies also requires that your client is stable and not actively at risk, psychotic or unstable. Soul therapies can be very powerful, so your client must be in a position where they can manage and cope with such changes as they are happening. Therefore, making your client aware of the power of such interventions and to be able to manage these appropriately is essential. Any therapist who offers soul therapies should take this into consideration. When soul therapies are being used in addition to your therapeutic work, if possible, it is advisable to work collaboratively with the other practitioner and discuss timings of any planned intervention so that you are not overloading your client with too much at any given time.

Summary

- Both EMDR and HLP use a three-pronged strategy working on past, current and future challenges. HLP understands past, current and future challenges as opportunities to learn and experience life lessons which increases client's awareness and understanding of what these challenges represent to them on their individual journey. The greater their understanding, the more effective clients will be at managing current and future challenges.
- The ideas of HLP can be incorporated within EMDR supervision, supporting supervisees to reflect on what their clients or organisations are mirroring back to them that may facilitate their own learning, growth and healing.
- It is imperative to take into account cultural considerations and make adaptations to the EMDR protocol when working with your clients, as well as adopting an anti-oppressive approach to clinical practice.
- Working online with clients can enable you to reach clients across the globe. However, it is important to be aware of how working online may impact your energy levels, especially if you are highly sensitive. Take steps to make sure you participate in regular self-care and grounding techniques.
- There are a number of ways to work at a spiritual or energetic level with children. Be creative and open to such ideas and work safely within their support system. Ideas include using crystals, sound therapy, aromatherapy, mantras, prayers, etc.
- Neurodiverse clients may have many traits that overlap with also being a highly sensitive, spiritual person. They can be highly attuned to energies and spiritual healing approaches.
- It is worth asking clients about past, current or planned psychedelic substance use. EMDR can be a wonderful therapy to prepare and resource clients for psychedelic experiences and can also facilitate the integration afterwards.
- It is important that clients have a degree of stability and insight to engage with the concepts of spirituality and HLP. It may not be appropriate for clients who are highly dissociative, unstable, at high levels of risk or have complex fragile personalities.

Afterword

'I know you are tired but come, this is the way.'

Rumi

Whilst writing the book, I debated whether to share much of my own personal story, exploring what the benefits would be and for most of the time I decided against it. I have been open about my past traumas and challenges in trainings as well as in my previous book (Dent, 2020) and have spent many years clearing and healing soul-level blocks and restrictions from this life and past lives. My primary life lesson is faith, specifically in relationships, which impacts me in all types of relationships including with myself and I have had a number of joint life lessons with key individuals as well as a variety of everyday and systemic life lessons to work through. Thankfully, I have a very strong spiritual faith which has been my guiding light. My past doesn't define me as it used to and I feel more at peace within myself although this is still something I am working through.

I was brought up as a Catholic in a predominantly white, judgemental environment in the south of England. From my perspective, we sadly continue to live in a very judgemental world. Most of us naturally and spontaneously form judgements by what we see, hear and sense about individuals and our surroundings which can very quickly shape our opinion, impression and influence or behaviour. It's not that forming judgements are necessarily the key issue because they happen, whether we are conscious of it or not. To me, the biggest challenge is noticing, acknowledging, and owning our judgements and learning how to release them from our heart space without acting on them.

My positionality in relation to this book is of a white, middle-aged, heterosexual, cisgender, neurodiverse, educated, spiritual but non-religious, able-bodied woman with a history of trauma and psychological difficulties (both personal, inter-generational and ancestral). I fully appreciate and recognise that my positionality has afforded me a great deal of privilege and power during my life. I have tried never to abuse this position, and if I have, to commit to repairing and healing any wrongdoing.

Currently in society, there appears to be such a strong desire to fit people into boxes, to separate and divide based on a whole host of different factors including colour, faith, gender, nationality, class and so forth. When such assumptions are made, we believe that a person represents those categories we, or maybe they, have put themselves in rather than connecting at a deeper, energetic level. I feel some of the above categories hold a great deal of shame to me because they come with a history from generations before where so much wrong, pain and suffering was caused. At a soul level, I resonate much more with Eastern beliefs and traditions. I feel most at peace imagining myself dancing around a fire in an American Indian community to the sound of drums, or sitting on a mountain side meditating in the Himalayas.

One of my core wounds, to which most of my triggers take me to, is that I have never felt I fitted in. Since early childhood I haven't felt a strong connection to my environment, Catholicism, ancestors and some peers and this is something I've battled with all my life. I am grateful that I have always felt a strong spiritual connection to a loving Divine Source, God, other deities and nature but I have struggled to settle in a world that can feel so devastatingly sad, cruel, unkind, uncompassionate and unloving at times. I also struggle with the disparity between what some people say and their actions or behaviour. Of course, there are areas where there is beauty and love but on the whole, people don't always appear to be very kind to each other. From my spiritual perspective though, we are all one and the same. I am not trying to ignore difference and diversity, but when we hold a transpersonal view, it allows us to move from a place of needing to be somebody to nobody to everybody (Dispenza, 2017). When you consider this approach and find a place of self-love within, the thought of hurting another person seems unthinkable because you are literally hurting yourself and not having self-love. Many of the times I have made mistakes in my life is because I have been hurting inside. It is easier to project onto others than to go within and work through the inner wounds and heal them.

My deepest core wound is 'I can't handle it anymore,' and there are times when I don't even want to handle it, it's all too much! This wound feels existential, really grappling with my past trauma history, both in this incarnation and many, many past lives, as well as my experience of being a human in the world. I would consider myself a strong, determined, soul who is completely committed to my soul mission and purpose. I have had plenty of opportunities to be with this wound and when it surfaces now, after a period of time battling with a situation or challenge, I imagine myself sitting down in protest to the Divine and saying, 'enough is enough.' I then raise my hands, turned upwards in front of me and surrender the burden to the Divine. The conversation roughly goes like this:

Me: 'You clearly know what you are doing, I'm exhausted and at breaking point and have had enough. I am just surrendering everything over to you and trusting in you.'
Divine: 'Thank you. Well done for trusting and surrendering.'

Sometimes the response feels cheekier:

> Divine: 'It took you long enough, now can you please step out of your own way and allow us support you!'

That's where transformative change happens. By letting go, surrendering and trusting, I am allowing myself to have faith in the Divine as well as myself. Within a short space of time, various things start happening, synchronicities etc. that help me to heal and regain strength to continue.

My natural default position is to hide away in a tiny part of the world and just be immersed in nature, as that is where I feel most at peace. The world to me can feel incredibly unsafe; where one is too scared to say or do something in case you will be judged and possibly openly ridiculed if you say the wrong thing, thus creating a feeling of living on egg shells. It has not passed my awareness of the irony that I also find my soul encouraging me to speak and write about such a triggering topic of spirituality which may make some feel uncomfortable. In writing this book, I am very clear that I am not suggesting individuals agree with my perspective, but instead consider finding their own authentic heart-based truth that, hopefully, has decent loving values. Perhaps this will enable us as a society to reach a place of tenderness, tolerance, connection and compassion to embrace living and working within difference and find the beauty and richness it brings. To own our own wounds and be prepared to work through them rather than fire them at another because we disagree. To treat each other as we would like to be treated ourselves with respect, dignity and humility. To recognise that others may represent a reflection of ourselves.

One of the most profound Divine experiences I was fortunate to participate in was at a spiritual retreat in 2023 with the world-renowned mantra singers Deva Premal and Miten. They had decided to hold a gathering in North Yorkshire, England as they practised for their forthcoming European tour. Seventy individuals from around the globe gathered to sing, meditate and dance for three days together in beautiful surroundings and company. The healing energy created was immense and electric but perhaps the most sacred of moments was when we were gathered for a Sufi dance. We were taught the words and the dance moves and then took our places opposite a partner as the music began and we started singing the song and dancing to the movements. We were instructed to look into the eyes of our partners and I gazed into the eyes of the person opposite me. The connection of pure unconditional Divine love I felt towards a complete stranger was incredible and I sensed they felt the same. Our eyes filled with tears that flowed down our cheeks as we held that gaze, and for those few precious moments nothing else mattered; we just felt pure unconditional Divine love. All differences dissolved as we transcended into an energy of oneness. We both then moved on to share a similar sensation when dancing with other partners and the tears continued to flow. The mixture of set, setting and the rhythmic bilateral movements of the beautiful Sufi dance was like nothing I had encountered before and will remain with me as a powerful internal resource forever. I know it is possible to feel Divine love for others, I just hope one day that more and more of us can find that connection in many areas of our lives. I believe that heart energy will become the most important form of global currency in years to come. I also believe that when we can strive towards this place, the world will become a kinder, safer, more accepting and loving place to live in harmony. It also goes without saying, remaining humble in our work and lives is also crucial.

With Divine love and light,
Alexandra, 2024

References

Abdul-Hamid, W.K., & Hacker Hughes, J. (2015). Integration of religion and spirituality into trauma psychotherapy: An example in Sufism? *Journal of EMDR Practice and Research*, 9(3), 150–156.

Abrams, H. (2008). Towards an understanding of mindful practices with children and adolescents in residential treatment. *Residential Treatment for Children & Youth*, 24 (1–2), 93–109.

Aggs, C., & Bambling, M. (2010). Teaching mindfulness to psychotherapists in clinical practice: The mindful therapy programme. *Counselling and Psychotherapy Research*, 10(4), 278–286.

American Psychiatric Association (1994) *Diagnostic and Statistical Manual of Mental Disorders: DSM-IV*. Washington, DC: American Psychiatric Association.

Armour, J.A. (1991). Anatomy and function of the intrathoracic neurons regulating the mammalian heart. In I.H. Zucker & J.P. Gilmore (Eds.), *Reflex control of the circulation* (pp. 1–37). Boca Raton, FL: CRC Press.

Armour, J.A. (2008). Potential clinical relevance of the 'little brain' on the mammalian heart. *Experimental Physiology*, 93(2): 165–176.

Artigas, L., Jarero, I., Mauer, M., López Cano, T., & Alcalá, N. (2000). *EMDR and traumatic stress after natural disasters: Integrative Treatment protocol and the Butterfly Hug*. Poster presentation, EMDRIA Conference, Toronto, Ontario, Canada, September 2000.

Beck, C.J., & Smith, S.A. (1993). *Nothing special: Living Zen*. New York: HarperCollins.

Botkins, A.L. (2000). The induction of after-death communications utilizing eye-movement desensitisation and reprocessing: A new discovery. *The Journal of Near Death Studies*, 18(3), 181–209.

Braud, W., & Anderson, R. (1998). *Transpersonal research methods for the social sciences*. Thousand Oaks, CA: Sage.

Braud, W., & Anderson, R. (2002). *Integral research skills study guide*. Palo Alto, CA: Institute of Transpersonal Psychology.

Brayer, R. (2023). *The art and science of EMDR: Helping clinicians bridge the path from protocol to practice*. Eau Claire, WI: PESI Publishing.

Brown, K.W., & Ryan, R.M. (2003). The benefits of being present: Mindfulness and its role in psychological wellbeing. *Journal of Personality and Social Psychology*, 84(4), 822–848.

Campbell, J. (2012). *The hero with a thousand faces (The collected works of Joseph Campbell)* (3rd ed.). Novato, CA: New World Library.

Caplan, M. (2009). *Eyes wide open: Cultivating discernment on the spiritual path.* Boulder, CO: Sounds True.

Childre, D., & McCraty, R. (2002). Psychological correlates of spiritual experience. *Biofeedback,* 29(4), 13–17.

Chopra, D. (1996). *The seven spiritual laws of success: A practical guide to the fulfilment of your dreams.* New York: Bantam Press.

Dent, A. (2020). *Using spirituality in psychotherapy: The heart led approach to clinical practice.* Abingdon: Routledge.

Dent, A. (2021). Heart-led psychotherapy: A biopsychosociospiritual model for clinical practice. *Transpersonal Psychology Review,* 23(1), 20–31.

Dispenza, J. (2017). *Becoming supernatural: How common people are doing the uncommon.* Carlsbad, CA: Hay House Inc.

Dobo, A.J. (2015). *Unburdening souls at the speed of thought: Psychology, Christianity, and the transforming power of EMDR.* Melbourne, FL: Soul Psych Publishers.

Dobo, A.J. (2023). *The hero's journey: Integrating Jungian psychology and EMDR therapy.* Melbourne, FL: Soul Psych Publishers.

Doyle, O. (2014). *Mindfulness plain and simple. A practical guide to peace through mindfulness.* London: Orion Publishing.

Dyer, W.W. (2013). *Stop the excuses!: How to change lifelong thoughts.* London: Hay House.

Elsaesser, E., Roe, C.A., Cooper, C.E., & Lorimer, D. (2020). Investigation of the phenomenology and impact of spontaneous and direct After-Death Communications (ADCs): Research findings. https://www.adcrp.org/_files/ugd/625c5c_9a9c095577914f2e9443d0fcb2021af9.pdf

Engel, G.L. (1977). The need for a new medical model: A challenge for biomedicine. *Science,* 196(4286), 129–136.

Golding, K.S. (2008). *Nurturing attachments: Supporting children who are fostered or adopted:*London & Philadelphia: Jessica Kingsley Publishers.

Gonzalez, A., Mosquera, D., & Fisher, J. (2012). Trauma processing in structural dissociation. In A. Gonzalez, & D. Mosquera (Eds.), *EMDR and dissociation: The progressive approach.* (1st ed.). A.I.

Grof, S., & Grof, C. (2010). *Holotropic breathwork: A new approach to self-exploration and therapy.* Albany, NY: SUNY Press.

Hacker Hughes, J. (2017). Towards a biopsychosociospiritual approach to psychological distress. *Transpersonal Psychology Review,* 19(1), 12–14.

Happy Buddha, The (2015). *Mindfulness and compassion: Embracing life with loving-kindness.* Brighton: Leaping Hare Press.

Hayes, S.C., Strosahl, K.D., & Wilson, K.G. (2016). *Acceptance and commitment therapy, The process and practice of mindful change* (2nd ed.). New York: Guilford Press.

Howe, L. (2010). *How to read the Akashic Records. Accessing the archive of the soul and its journey.* Boulder, CO: Sounds True.

Hughes, D.A. (2007). *Attachment-focused family therapy.* New York & London: W.W. Norton & Co.

Ingerman, S. (2014). *Walking in light: The everyday empowerment of a shamanic life.* Boulder, CO: Sounds True.

Irving, J.A., Dobkin, P.L., & Park, J. (2009). Cultivating mindfulness in HCPs: A review of empirical studies of mindfulness-based stress reduction (MBSR). *Complementary Therapies in Clinical Practice,* 15(2), 61–66.

Ivtzan, I., & Lomas, T. (2016). *Mindfulness in positive psychology: The science of meditation and wellbeing.* London & New York: Routledge.

Jarero, I., Artigas, L., Uribe, S., & Miranda, A. (2014). EMDR therapy humanitarian trauma recovery interventions in Latin America and the Caribbean. *Journal of EMDR Practice and Research,* 8(4), 260–268.

Johari, H. (2000). *Chakras: Energy centres of transformation.* Rochester, VT: Destiny Books.

Jung, C.G. (1959a). *The archetypes and the collective unconscious* (G. Adler & R.F.C. Hull, Eds. & Trans.). In The collected works of C.G. Jung, Vol. 9, Part I. Bollingen Series XX. Princeton, NJ: Princeton University Press.

Kabat-Zinn, J. (1982). An out-patient program in behavioural medicine for chronic pain patients based on the practice of mindfulness meditation: Theoretical considerations and preliminary results. *General Hospital Psychiatry,* 4(1), 33–47.

Kabat-Zinn, J. (1994). *Wherever you go, there you are. Mindfulness meditation in everyday life.* New York: Hyperion.

Kabat-Zinn, J., Lipworth, L., Burncy, R. & Sellers, W. (1986). Four year follow-up of a meditation-based program for the self-regulation of chronic pain: Treatment outcomes and compliance. *The Clinical Journal of Pain,* 2(3), 159.

Kennedy, A. (2014). Compassion-focused EMDR. *Journal of EMDR Practice and Research,* (8)3, 135–146.

Khan, M. (2023). *Working within diversity: A reflective guide to anti-oppressive practice in counselling and therapy.* London & Philadelphia: Jessica Kingsley Publishers.

Kilrea, K.A., Taylor, S., Bilodeau, C., Wittman, M., Gutiérrez, D.L., & Kübel, S.L. (2023). Measuring an ongoing state of wakefulness: The development and validation of the inventory of secular/spiritual wakefulness (WAKE). *Journal of Humanistic Psychology,* 1–32. doi:10.1177/00221678231185891

King, D.E. (2000). *Faith, spirituality and medicine: Toward the making of a healing practitioner.* Binghamton, NY: Haworth Pastoral Press.

Knipe, J. (2015). *EMDR toolbox: Theory and treatment of complex PTSD and dissociation.* New York: Springer Publishing Company.

Korn, D.L., & Leeds, A.M. (2002). Preliminary evidence of efficacy for EMDR resource development and installation in the stabilization phase of treatment of complex post traumatic disorder. *Journal of Clinical Psychology,* 58(12), 1465–1487.

Krystal, S., Prendergast, J., Krystal, P., Fenner, P., Shapiro, I., & Shapiro, K. (2002). Transpersonal psychology, eastern nondual philosophy, and EMDR. In F. Shapiro (Ed.), *EMDR as an integrative psychotherapy approach: Experts of diverse orientations explore the paradigm prism* (pp. 319–339). Washington, DC: American Psychological Association.

Laszlo, E. (2007). *Science and the Akashic field: An integral theory of everything* (2nd ed.). Rochester, VT: Inner Traditions.

Laszlo, E. (2009). *The Akashic experience: Science and the cosmic memory field.* Rochester, VT: Inner Traditions.

Leeds, A.M. (1998). Lifting the burden of shame: Using EMDR resource installation to resolve a therapeutic impasse. In P. Manfield (Ed.), *Extending EMDR: A case book of innovative applications* (pp. 256–282). New York: W.W. Norton & Co.

Linehan, M.M. (1993). *Skills training manual for treating borderline personality disorder.* New York & London: Guilford Press.

Logie, R.D.J., Bowers, M., Dent, A., Elliott, J., O'Connor, M., Russell, A. (2020). *Using stories in EMDR: A guide to the storytelling (narrative) approach in EMDR therapy.* Frome: Trauma Aid UK.

Logie, R.D.J., & De Jongh, A. (2014). The 'flashforwards procedure': Confronting the catastrophe. *Journal of EMDR Practice and Research,* 8(1), 25–32.

Lovett, J. (1999). *Small wonders: Healing childhood trauma with EMDR.* New York: The Free Press.

Lovett, J. (2015). *Trauma-attachment tangle. Modifying EMDR to help children resolve trauma and develop loving relationships.* New York & London: Routledge.

MacLean, C.A. (2003). Transpersonal dimensions in healing pre/perinatal trauma with EMDR (Eye Movement Desensitization and Reprocessing). *Journal of Prenatal & Perinatal Psychology & Health,* 18(1), 39–70.

McClintock, C.H. (2015). Opening the heart: A spirituality of gratitude. *Spirituality in Clinical Practice,* 2(1), 21–22.

McCraty, R. (2003). *Heart-brain neurodynamics: The making of emotions.* Boulder Creek, CA: Institute of HeartMath.

McCraty, R., Atkinson, M., Tomasino, D. & Tiller, W.A. (1998). The electricity of touch: Detection and measurement of cardiac energy exchange between two people. In K.H. Pribam (Ed.), *Brain and values: Is biological science of values possible?* (pp. 259–379). Mahwah, NJ: Lawrence Erlbaum Associates.

McKee, D.D., & Chappel, J.N. (1992). Spirituality and medical practice. *Journal of Family Practice,* 35(201), 205–208.

Marich, J., & Dansiger, S. (2017). *EMDR therapy and mindfulness for trauma-focused care.* New York: Springer Publishing Company.

Mbazzi, F.B., Dewally, A., Admasu, K., Duagani, Y., Wamala, K., Vera, A., Bwesigye, D., and Roth, G. (2021). Cultural adaptations of the standard EMDR protocol in five African countries. *Journal of EMDR Practice and Research,* 15(1), 29–43.

Mehrotra, S. (2014). Humanitarian projects and growth of EMDR therapy in Asia. *Journal of EMDR Practice and Research,* 8(4), 252–259.

Miller, R. (2011). The feeling-state theory of behavioural and substance addictions and the feeling-state addiction protocol. https://emdrtherapyvolusia.com/wp-content/up loads/2016/12/Feeling-State_Addiction_Protocol.pdf

Mother, The (1972). *Collected Works of the Mother,* Vol. *16* (p. 247). Pondicherry: Sri Aurobindo Ashram Trust.

Napoli, M., Krech, P., & Holley, L. (2005). Mindfulness training for elementary school students: The attention academy. *Journal of Applied School Psychology,* 21(1), 99–125.

National Institute for Health and Care Excellence (2022). NICE Guideline, Depression in adults: Recognition and management. https://www.nice.org.uk/guidance/ng222

Newton, M. (2011). *Journey of souls: Case studies of life between lives.* Woodbury, MN: Llewellyn Publications.

Norcross, J.C., & Lambert, M.J. (2018). Psychotherapy relationships that work III. *Psychotherapy,* 55(4), 303–315.

O'Malley, A.G. (2018). *Sensorimotor-focused EMDR: A new paradigm for psychotherapy and peak performance.* London & New York: Routledge.

O'Malley, A.G. (2024). Quantum EMDR (QEMDR); A guide for EMDR therapists. *The Science of Psychotherapy,* 12(1), 42–71.

O'Shea, K. (2009). The EMDR Early Trauma Protocol. In Shapiro, R (Eds.), *EMDR solutions II: For depression, eating disorders, performance and more* (pp.313–334). New York: W.W. Norton & Co.

Parnell, L. (1996). Eye movement desensitization and reprocessing (EMDR) and spiritual unfolding. *The Journal of Transpersonal Psychology*, 28(2), 129–153. http://www.atpweb.org/jtparchive/trps-28-96-02-129.pdf

Parnell, L. (2007). *A therapist's guide to EMDR: Tools and techniques for successful treatment.* New York & London: W.W. Norton & Co.

Parnell, L. (2008). *Tapping in: A step-by-step guide to activating your healing resources through bilateral stimulation.* Boulder, CO: Sounds True.

Powell, A. (2018). *Conversations with the soul. A psychiatrist reflects: Essays on life, death and beyond.* London: Muswell Hill Press.

Radin, D., Hayssen, G., Emoto, M., & Kizu, T. (2006). Double-blind test of the effects of distant intention on water crystal formation. *Explore*, 2(5), 408–411.

Raine-Smith, H., & Rose, J. (2025). *Psychedelic-assisted EMDR therapy: A memory-consolidation approach to psychedelic healing.* London: Routledge.

Read, T. (2019). *Walking shadows: Archetype and psyche in crisis and growth.* London: Aeon Books Ltd.

Rosch, P.J., & Markov, M.S. (2004). *Bioelectromagnetic medicine.* Boca Raton, FL: CRC Press.

Segal, Z.V., Williams, J.M.G., & Teasdale, J.D. (2002). *Mindfulness-based cognitive therapy for depression: A new approach to preventing relapse.* New York: Guilford Press.

Shapiro, F. (2001). *Eye Movement Desensitisation and Reprocessing. Basic principles, protocols and procedures* (2nd ed.). New York: Guilford Press.

Shapiro, F. (2018). *Eye Movement Desensitisation and Reprocessing (EMDR) therapy: Basic principles, protocols, and procedures* (3rd ed.). New York & London: Guilford Press.

Shapiro, R. (2005). *EMDR solutions: Pathways to healing.* New York: W.W. Norton & Co.

Shapiro, R. (2009). *EMDR solutions II: For depression, eating disorders, performance and more.* New York: W.W. Norton & Co.

Shapiro, S., & Carlson, L. (2009). *The art and science of mindfulness: Integrating mindfulness into psychology and the helping professions.* Washington, DC: American Psychological Association.

Shapiro, S., de Sousa, S., & Jazaieri, H. (2016). Mindfulness, mental health and positive psychology. In I. Ivtzan & T. Lomas (Eds.). (2016). *Mindfulness in positive psychology* (pp. 108–125). London & New York: Routledge.

Siegel, D. (2010). *The mindful therapist: A clinician's guide to mindsight and neural integration.* New York: W.W. Norton & Co.

Siegel, I.R. (2013). Therapist as a container for spiritual resonance and client transformation within transpersonal psychotherapy: An exploratory heuristic study. *The Journal of Transpersonal Psychology*, 45(1), 49–74.

Siegel, I.R. (2017). *The sacred path of the therapists: Modern healing, ancient wisdom, and client transformation.* New York & London: W.W. Norton & Co.

Siegel, I.R. (2018). EMDR as a transpersonal therapy: A trauma-focused approach to awakening consciousness. *Journal of EMDR Practice and Research*, 12(1), 24–43.

Siegel, I.R. (2019). Spontaneous awakening in transpersonal psychology. *The Journal of Transpersonal Psychology*, 51(2), 198–224.

Silva, R.C., Martini, P., Hohoff, C., Mattevi, S., Bortolomasi, M., Menesello, V., Gennarelli, M., Baune, B., & Minelli, A. (2024). DNA methylation changes in association with trauma-focused psychotherapy efficacy in treatment-resistant depression patients: a prospective longitudinal study. *European Journal of Psychotraumatology*, 15(1), 2314913. doi:10.1080/20008066.2024.2314913

Sorrell, M. (2019). *The wonder of stillness: Meditation for children. A practical guide for parents and teachers*. Stillness Publishing.

Spierings, J. (2004). *Working with EMDR in the treatments of clients with other (sub) cultures and religions: Multi-culti EMDR*. Paper presented at the 5th EMDR Europe Association Conference, Stockholm, Sweden.

Sulmasy, D.P. (2002). A biopsychosocial-spiritual model for the care of patients at the end of life. *The Gerontologist*, 42, Special Issue III, 24–33.

Taylor, S. (2017). *The leap: The psychology of spiritual awakening*. London: Hay House.

Taylor, S. (2019). Spontaneous awakening experiences. Beyond religion and spiritual practice. *The Journal of Transpersonal Psychology,44*(1), 73–91.

Taylor, S., & Egeto-Szabo, K. (2017). Exploring awakening experiences in terms of their triggers, characteristics, duration and side-effects. *The Journal of Transpersonal Psychology*, 49(1), 45–65.

Teilhard de Chardin, P. (1975). *The human phenomenon*. New York: Harper and Row.

Tinker, R.H., & Wilson, S.A. (1999). *Through the eyes of a child: EMDR with children*. New York: W.W.Norton & Company.

Tolle, E. (2005). *The power of now: A guide to spiritual enlightenment*. London: Hodder Mobius.

Tomlinson, A. (2012). *Healing the eternal soul: Insights from past life and spiritual regression*. Fleetwood: From the Heart Press.

Van der Kolk, B. (2014). *The body keeps the score: Brain, mind, and body in the healing of trauma*. New York: Penguin Books.

Villoldo, A. (2005). *Mending the past and healing the future with soul retrieval*. London: Hay House.

Vinkers, C.H., Geuze, E., van Rooij, S.J.H., Kennis, M., Schür, R.R., Nispeling, D.M., Smith, A.K., Nievergelt, C.M., Uddin, M., Rutten, B.P.F., Vermetten, E., & Boks, M.P. (2021). Successful treatment of post-traumatic stress disorder reverses DNA methylation marks. *Molecular Psychiatry*, 26(4), 1264–1271.

Walsh, R., & Vaughan, F. (1993). On transpersonal definitions. *Journal of Transpersonal Psychology*, 25(2), 125–182.

Watts, F. (2018). Psychology, religion and the transpersonal. *Transpersonal Psychology Review*, 20(1), 15–22.

Weiss, B., & Weiss, A. (2012). *Miracles happen: The transformational healing power of past life memories*. London: Hay House.

White, R.A. (1994). *Exceptional human experience: Background papers*. Dix Hills, NY: EHE Network.

Wilber, K. (2000). *Integral psychology: Consciousness, spirit, psychology, therapy*. Boulder, CO: Shambhala Publications.

Williams, M., & Penman, D. (2011). *Mindfulness: A practical guide to finding peace in a frantic world*. London: Piatkus.

Williams, M., & Penman, D. (2023). *Deeper mindfulness: The new way to rediscover calm in a chaotic world*. London: Piatkus.

WHOQOL SRPB Group (2006). A cross-cultural study of spirituality, religion, and personal beliefs as components of quality of life. *Social Science and Medicine*, 62(6), 1486–1497.

World Health Organization (2013). *Guidelines for the management of conditions specifically related to stress.* Geneva: World Health Organization.

Zenner, C., Herrnleben-Kurz, S., & Walach, H. (2014). Mindfulness-based interventions in schools – a systemic review and meta-analysis. *Frontiers in Psychology*, 5, 603.

Zoogman, S., Goldberg, S., Hoyt, W., & Miller, L. (2014). Mindfulness interventions with youth: A meta-analysis. *Mindfulness*, 6(2), 1–13.

Websites

www.dharma.org

A website offering information about insight meditation tradition and retreats.

www.drirenesiegel.com

Information about classes, workshops, retreats and online distance learning courses, integrating psychotherapy with shamanic healing.

www.emdrassociation.org.uk

The official UK EMDR website offering information about training, resources, finding EMDR accredited practitioners and consultants, courses and conferences.

www.thefourwinds.com

Information on the world's renowned school of energy medicine, offering retreats, online training, resources etc.

www.franticworld.com

The website that accompanies Mark Williams and Danny Penman's book, with links to further meditations and books, upcoming talks, events and retreats. Also has a forum in which you can discuss experiences and share these with others.

www.gaiahouse.co.uk

Meditation retreat centre offering silent meditation retreats with a Buddhist tradition.

www.headspace.com

Online support on how to learn to meditate with resources for children and adults.

www.heartledpsychotherapy.com

The official HLP website.

www.heartmath.com

For information on Heartmath technology, training, coaching, research etc.

Index

For Product Safety Concerns and Information please contact our EU
representative GPSR@taylorandfrancis.com
Taylor & Francis Verlag GmbH, Kaufingerstraße 24, 80331 München, Germany

9 781032 834993